Calorie Counter

Calorie Counter

PARRAGON

This edition published and distributed
by Parragon, 1999

Parragon
13 Whiteladies Road
Clifton, Bristol BS8 1PB

Produced by Magpie Books, an imprint of
Robinson Publishing Ltd, London

ISBN 0–75252–988–9

A copy of the British Library Cataloguing-in-Publication Data is available from the British Library

Important Note

The publishers and author cannot accept liability for any injury or loss to any person acting or refraining from action as a result of the material in this book. Before commencing a diet or any health treatment, always consult your own doctor.

Printed and bound in the EC

Contents

INTRODUCTION

Introduction

How to use this book

• Read through the following sections and make sure you understand the importance of a balanced diet and the principles underlying successful weight loss.

• Compare your weight with the information on pages 16 and 17 and decide if you are overweight. Remember, these tables are based on average weights for men and women and it is quite possible to be lighter or heavier than the weight shown for your height and still be perfectly healthy. If you are in any doubt about whether or not to lose weight, consult your doctor.

• Using the table on page 9, calculate how long it will take you to lose any extra weight if you were to lose (a) 1 lb (454g) each week, (b) 2 lbs (907g) each week. Decide what your weight loss goal will be.

• Examine your current diet and lifestyle and decide what improvements need to be made. Look at the charts on page 5 to determine your daily Calorie requirements. Ask yourself whether you eat more or less than the recommended amount. Think about *when* you eat. Do you snack frequently during the day, for example, or while watching television? If so, see the chart on page 13, which compares the fat and Calorie contents of some common snacks with some alternative food choices. Do you eat high-fat, high-calorie snack foods because you are always in a hurry or too tired to cook a proper meal? Do you eat when you are feeling bored or frustrated? Asking these questions may help you make changes to your current eating habits, and in the long term this will help you lose weight.

• Look in your refrigerator and cupboards. Which foods are high in fat and high in Calories? Perhaps you could get rid of these straight away. Could you replace them with more healthy alternatives?

• Read the information in the sections on **Tips for reducing your fat intake** (page 12) and **Tips for reducing your sugar intake** (page 15).

• Use the Calorie and fat counter on pages 31–126 to help you plan well-balanced, low-calorie, low-fat meals.

• Try some of the recipes on pages 127–138.

• Use the menu planners on pages 141–154 to plan a new, more healthy diet.

The importance of a healthy diet

A healthy diet is one that contains a wide variety of foods and includes protein, carbohydrate and fat, as well as vitamins and minerals.

Protein is essential for the growth, repair and maintenance of cells and is found in foods such as meat, fish, eggs, milk, dairy produce, beans and nuts.

Carbohydrate is a valuable energy source. There are two forms: complex carbohydrates (found in foods such as cereals, potatoes, rice, pasta and bread) and simple carbohydrates (basically sugars, found in foods such as chocolate, biscuits, ice cream and soft drinks, as well as in fruit). Complex carbohydrates are better for us because as well as energy they provide plenty of fibre, which is essential for a healthy digestive system and may help lower cholesterol levels in the blood.

Important vitamins, minerals and fibre found in complex carbohydrate foods are rarely found in simple carbohydrates, which are sometimes described as providing "empty Calories".

Fats are needed to help insulate and protect the body and are a concentrated source of energy. There are two main types of fat: saturated fats (found in meat, dairy products, cooking fat, biscuits and pastries) and unsaturated fats (found in foods such as olive oil, polyunsaturated spreads, sunflower oil and oily fish).

Why we need Calories

The term "Calorie" (also known as kilocalorie) refers to the kind of energy we get from food. Our bodies need energy in order to function properly – to help us move, exercise and play, for example, and to help us maintain a stable body temperature. Even while we are sleeping the cells in our bodies use energy for growth and repair.

All foods provide energy – including liquid foods such as milk, fruit juices and alcohol. The only liquid food that does not contain energy is water. Water contains *no* Calories at all. Proteins, carbohydrates and fats each provide different amounts of energy. One gram (0.035 oz) of protein provides our bodies with four Calories, as does one gram of carbohydrate. However, one gram of fat provides nine Calories – more than twice the amount of energy derived from proteins or carbohydrates.

Each year, using a process known as caliometry, new foods are tested to see how many Calories they contain. We now know how many Calories there are in thousands of different foods. The Calorie and fat contents listed in the Calorie counter in this book were derived from the food labels of a variety of foods sold in high-street supermarkets and from *The Composition of Foods* (fifth edition, 1991) by permission of The Royal Society of Chemistry and Her Majesty's Stationery Office.

How many Calories do we need?

The number of Calories we need each day differs between individuals – some people need lots, others a relatively small number. Pregnant women, for example, need more Calories to generate the extra energy needed by their growing bodies and their developing babies, and a very active person needs more Calories than someone with a sedentary lifestyle. Men tend to require more Calories than women because their bodies are bigger. An average man needs about 2800 Calories a day; an average woman needs about 2100. A pregnant woman requires around 2350 Calories a day. If breastfeeding, she needs around 2750. Both men and women need more Calories when taking part in physical activity, especially when it involves heavy manual labour. The table on page 5 shows the recommended daily Calorie requirements for men and women aged 18–64 with both sedentary and active lifestyles.

How much fat do we need?

For health reasons it is recommended that no more

Daily Calorie Requirements

Men

Age	Lifestyle	Daily Calorie Requirements
18–34	Sedentary	2500
	Moderately active	2900
	Active	3350
35–64	Sedentary	2400
	Moderately active	2750
	Active	3350

Daily Calorie Requirements

Women

Age	Lifestyle	Daily Calorie Requirements
18–34	Sedentary	2000
	Moderately active	2100
	Active	2500
35–64	Sedentary	2000
	Moderately active	2100
	Active	2500

than 30 per cent of our total energy intake is derived from fat. This means that if you have a diet of 2000 Calories a day, for example, no more than 600 of these Calories should come from fat.

It is also recommended that we consume unsaturated fats rather than saturated fats. This is because saturated fats are associated with increased levels of cholesterol in the blood and a higher risk of coronary heart disease, whereas unsaturated fats can help to reduce the levels of cholesterol in the blood and may help prevent heart disease. The two kinds of unsaturated fats seen on food labels, monounsaturated fats and polyunsaturated fats, are both a healthier option for you than saturated fats.

The table on the next page shows the characteristics of different types of fat, and the table on page 8 gives some of their common sources.

What happens when your Calorie intake is too high?

The body only uses those Calories it needs in order to function correctly. Any surplus Calories in the form of excess fats, proteins and carbohydrates are stored as fat in the body. So if you eat more Calories than your body needs you will put on weight; if you eat less than your body needs, you will lose weight. For example, if your energy requirements are 2000 Calories a day but you eat 2500 Calories, you will gain weight; if your requirements are 2500 Calories a day but you eat only 2000, you begin to lose weight.

Characteristics of fats

Saturated fats

- Are usually solid at room temperature.
- Are found mainly in foods of animal origin (such as butter).
- Are sometimes found in large amounts in vegetable products (such as coconut oil and palm oil).
- Are believed to be harmful to your health.
- Are not essential and can be removed entirely from your diet.

Monounsaturated fats

- Are liquid at room temperature.
- Are usually derived from plant sources (such as olive oil).
- Are found in some animal foods (such as herring and sardine oil).
- Are believed to be essential for your health.

Polyunsaturated fats

- Are usually liquid at room temperature.
- Are found mostly in plant sources (such as almond oil, corn oil and sunflower oil).
- Are found in some animal sources (such as fish).
- Are found in "polyunsaturated" margarines.
- Are essential to the diet. Some may even help to prevent heart disease. These are known as Omega-3 oils and are found in oily fish such as herrings, mackerel and sardines.

Sources of fat

Fats and oils	Saturated fat	Unsaturated fat Mono-	Poly-
Butter	68	23	4
Fat, beef	41	47	4
Fat, chicken	30	45	20
Fat, duck	29	57	13
Fat, lamb	52	41	5
Fat, pork	35	42	15
Lard	44	44	9
Margarine, hard	39	47	10
Margarine, "polyunsaturated"	17	27	52
Margarine, soft	30	41	26
Oil, almond	5	0	95
Oil, coconut	89	8	2
Oil, corn	13	25	58
Oil, herring	22	56	20
Oil, olive	14	73	12
Oil, palm	45	45	9
Oil, salmon	27	42	26
Oil, sardine	20	57	20
Oil, sesame	14	40	43
Oil, sunflower	12	33	58
Oil, tuna	19	41	38

Tips for successful weight loss

• Talk to your doctor. This is especially important for pregnant women, anyone who has just had a child, or anyone who may have an underlying condition that could be affected by diet. Find out whether you really are overweight and to what extent.

• Aim for gradual rather than sudden weight loss. Experts recommend you aim for weight loss of around 1–2 lb (454–907 g) a week. This is because evidence suggests that people who achieve slow, steady weight loss are more likely to remain at a lower weight than those who achieve sudden, drastic weight loss (which is usually short-lived). The table below shows the recommended daily Calorie intake for men and women wanting to lose 1–2 lb per week.

Daily Calorie intakes for gradual weight loss

Remember that this table is just a guide – Calorie requirements also vary according to age, weight and lifestyle.

	weekly weight loss		Calories per day
Men	1 lb	454 g	2300
Women	1 lb	454 g	1500
Men	2 lb	907 g	1700
Women	2 lb	907 g	1000

• Set a realistic target. It is more sensible to try dieting and taking regular exercise for two weeks followed by a review of your progress, than to tell yourself "I will live on grapefruit for the next three months". Remember, diets of less than 1000 Calories a day generally do more harm than good.

• Aim to lose weight by (a) reducing your Calorie intake (dieting to reduce the number of Calories you consume) and (b) increasing your energy expenditure (becoming more physically active in order to use up the Calories you consume and those stored as fat). The tables on pages 18 and 19 show the number of Calories used while taking part in various sporting and non-sporting activities. Use them to help you measure your energy expenditure through physical activity.

• Eat sensibly. The needs of your body do not change just because you are trying to lose weight. You still need protein, carbohydrate, vitamins, minerals and *some* fats. See page 20 for an explanation of the importance of vitamins and minerals, and pages 21–25 for examples of the kinds of foods in which these valuable chemicals can be found. The tables on pages 143–145 show the different food groups from which you should be selecting items for your diet.

• Drink plenty of water. In the early weeks of a diet you can lose weight quickly because your body easily loses excess fluids. Later, when weight loss is more difficult to achieve, don't be tempted to drink less in order to recreate this effect. Water is vital for your body to function properly and it contains no calories.

• Be accurate when weighing yourself. Set your

bathroom scales to zero and check they are working correctly by weighing a pre-weighed product (such as a pound of sugar). Always weigh yourself at the same time of day and preferably when you are not wearing any clothes.

• Avoid weighing yourself all the time. Your weight fluctuates daily, and there is really no need to weigh yourself more than once a week.

• Plan your meals. Try to eat small meals throughout the day rather than using up your full Calorie entitlement in one large meal. Eating small amounts regularly will lessen the chances of you feeling hungry and will help you to lose weight. If you eat a large evening meal shortly before going to bed your body has no chance to use up those Calories during daily activity.

• Read the sections on **Tips for reducing your fat intake** and **Tips for reducing your sugar intake** on pages 12–15.

Foods to avoid – a quick guide

Biscuits	Margarine
Butter	Mayonnaise
Cakes	Oily salad dressings
Chocolate	Puddings
Cooking oils	Sugar
Crisps	Sweetened drinks
Ice cream	Sweets

Tips for reducing your fat intake

- Replace butter or margarine with a reduced fat spread but *don't* use more of it simply because it's lower in Calories.
- If you prefer to use butter and margarine on bread, spread it thinly.
- Use semi-skimmed (half-fat) or skimmed (virtually fat-free) milk instead of whole (full-fat) milk.
- If you need to use cream, use less of it and use single cream rather than double cream.
- If you want to eat hard cheese, choose one that has a stronger flavour than your normal choice and use less of it.
- Try using half-fat hard cheese or even cottage cheese instead of full-fat hard cheese.
- Buy low-fat yoghurt or low-fat fromage frais and try using it instead of cream.
- Choose meats that are lower in fat such as chicken and turkey, instead of high-fat meats like pork and beef.
- Always choose the leanest cut of meat available and trim off any fat you can see.
- Because there is hidden fat in meat, eat less meat and more potatoes, vegetables and pulses.
- Use low-fat salad dressings instead of mayonnaise and salad cream.
- Cut down on biscuits, cakes, chocolate, crisps, and pastries. Find alternative, low-fat snacks.

- Bake, grill or steam food. Avoid fried foods.
- Replace high-fat snacks with low-fat snacks. Some examples are given below.

	Fat content per 100 grams
High-fat snack	
Almonds	55.8
Bombay mix	32.9
Brazil nuts	68.2
Cheddar cheese	34.4
Chocolate biscuits	27.6
Cream cheese	47.4
Crisps	37.6
Milk chocolate	30.3
Peanuts	46.1
Taramasalata	46.4
Low-fat snack	
Apple	0.1
Banana	0.3
Carrots	0.5
Celery	0.2
Chestnuts	2.7
Cottage cheese	3.9
Crispbread	2.1
Oranges	0.1
Pitta bread	1.2
Yoghurt, plain	3.0

- Avoid fast foods that are high in fat. Examples of some commonly available burgers are given below (the figures show what percentage of each product is fat). Remember, only 30 per cent of your total daily Calorie intake should come from fat.

Type of fast food	**Percentage of fat**
Burger King	
Cheeseburger	45
Double Cheeseburger	53
Whopper	55
Whopper with cheese	56
Double Whopper with cheese	59
McDonald's	
Hamburger	21
Cheeseburger	38
Quarter Pounder	45
Quarter Pounder with Cheese	51
Big Mac	50
Wendy's	
Hamburger (kid's)	33
Hamburger	38
Cheeseburger (kid's)	38
Double Hamburger, plain	46
Double hamburger (with everything)	48

Tips for reducing your sugar intake

- Avoid foods with a high sugar content (check the labels). Remember that sugar has many different forms and may be referred to as cane sugar, brown sugar, raw sugar, honey, muscovado or syrup.
- One of the best ways to cut down on sugar is to stop adding it to tea and coffee. If you cut your sugar intake by half (for example, by using one teaspoon of sugar instead of two) this will be an important contribution to your diet.
- Use less sugar when cooking. Buy ready-made low-sugar desserts.
- Buy fruit tinned in natural juice rather than syrup.
- Substitute sugar-coated cereals with plain cereals.
- Cut down on the number of biscuits, cakes, honey, jam, marmalade, syrup, sweet pastries and treacle you eat.
- Avoid all kinds of sweets and chocolates. Even cereal bars that claim to be "healthy" may be packed with sugar.
- Choose low-calorie soft drinks or unsweetened fruit juice diluted with water.
- Avoid eating large quantities of dried fruits. These "healthy" snacks are high in sugar and should be eaten sparingly.

How much should you weigh?

The following two tables show desirable weights for men and women aged 25 and over. Note, however, that the figures given are approximate and should be used only as a guide. Also, many people now argue that there is no such thing as a desirable weight.

Desirable weights for men

Height		Small frame		Medium frame		Large frame	
m	*ft in*	*kg*	*lb*	*kg*	*lb*	*kg*	*lb*
1.54	5 1	53	116	56	123.5	60.5	133.5
1.57	5 2	54	119	58	127	62	136.5
1.60	5 3	55.5	122	59	130	63.5	140
1.62	5 4	57	125	60.5	133	65	143.5
1.65	5 5	58.5	128.5	62	136.5	67	147
1.67	5 6	60	132.5	64	140.5	68	150.5
1.70	5 7	62	136.5	66	145	71	156.5
1.72	5 8	64	140.5	67.5	149	73	160.5
1.75	5 9	66	145	69.5	153	75	164.5
1.77	5 10	67.5	149	71.5	157.5	77	169
1.80	5 11	69.5	153	73.5	162	79	174
1.82	6 0	71	157	75.5	166.5	81	178.5
1.85	6 1	73	161.5	77	171	83	183.5
1.87	6 2	75	165.5	80	176	85.5	188.5
1.90	6 3	77	169.5	82	181	87.5	193

How much should you weigh?

Desirable weights for women

Height		Small frame		Medium frame		Large frame	
m	*ft in*	*kg*	*lb*	*kg*	*lb*	*kg*	*lb*
1.45	4 9	44.5	98	47	104	52	114
1.47	4 10	45.5	100	48.5	107	53	117
1.49	4 11	47	103	50	110	54.5	120
1.52	5 0	48	106	51	113	56	123
1.54	5 1	49.5	109	52.5	116	57	126
1.57	5 2	51	112	54.5	120	59	130
1.60	5 3	52	115	56	124	61	134
1.62	5 4	54	119	58	128	62.5	138
1.65	5 5	56	123	60	132	64.5	142
1.67	5 6	58	127	61.5	136	66	146
1.70	5 7	59.5	131	63.5	140	68	150
1.72	5 8	61	135	65	144	70	154
1.75	5 9	63	139	67	148	72	159
1.77	5 10	65	143	69	152	74.5	164
1.80	5 11	66.5	147	71	157	77	169

How much energy do you burn?

The table below shows how much energy you might burn on average during various physical activites, ranked according to the energy required. Figures are based on someone weighing 65 kilograms (10 st 2 lb). Heavier people usually need more energy than lighter people to complete the same activities.

Non-sporting activities

Activity	Cal/hour
Sleeping	60
Knitting	90
Sitting	90
Horse-riding, moderate	100
Driving a car	120
Writing	120
Typing	120
Piano playing	150
Gardening, weeding	210
House cleaning	240
Shopping	240
Walking, leisurely	240
Dancing, relaxed	380

Dancing, fast	410
Heavy manual work	450
Gardening, digging	480
Hill climbing	480
Hill climbing with a backpack	510
Climbing stairs	660

Sporting activities

Activity	Cal/hour
Cycling, gentle	240
Running, slow	280
Jogging	330
Skiing	390
Golf	390
Running, fast	400
Playing tennis	420
Weight training	420
Aerobics	430
Swimming, relaxed	510
Cycling, uphill	600
Playing squash	840

The importance of vitamins and minerals

Vitamins are chemicals that our bodies require in very small amounts. They each have a different function, and without them we would become ill. Although the body is able to make some of its own vitamins (such as vitamin D and vitamin K), most must be obtained from the foods we eat. This is also true of minerals, which, although required in even smaller quantities than vitamins, are essential to the way our bodies function.

Different vitamins and minerals are found in different foods, which is why it is important to maintain a varied diet. It is simply not possible to obtain all the vitamins and minerals the body needs from just one type of food.

The main vitamins and minerals and some of their food sources are listed on pages 21–25. Use this information to plan menus that will give you all the vitamins and minerals you need. Notice that the same vitamin or mineral may be obtained from a variety of different foods, which has the advantage that if you don't like oranges, for example, you can obtain your vitamin C from tomatoes or strawberries. Similarly, if you dislike milk, you can obtain your calcium from yoghurt.

Over the course of a week, your diet should include all the vitamins and minerals listed in the table.

Vitamin	Food sources (examples)	Deficiency results in
A (retinol)	Egg yolk Liver Milk Cabbage Carrots Lettuce	Eye problems
B_1 (thiamin)	Green vegetables Meat Nuts Soybeans Yeast	Beriberi (pain, swelling and paralysis of limbs)
B_2 (riboflavin)	Eggs Fish Green leafy vegetables Liver Milk Poultry Yeast	Eye problems Mouth sores
Niacin	Fish Green vegetables Lean meat Poultry Wholegrain bread Wholegrain cereal	Pellagra (diarrhoea, dematitis, nervous disorders)
B_6 (pyridoxine)	Meat Vegetables Wholegrain cereals	Deficiency is rare

Vitamin	Food sources (examples)	Deficiency results in
Pantothenic acid	Animal products Beans Cereals Peas	Deficiency is rare
Folic acid	Beans Cereals Eggs Liver Peas Raw leaf salads	Anaemia
B_{12} (cyanocobalamin)	Eggs Liver Milk	Anaemia Damage to nerve cells
Biotin	Cereals Egg yolk Fish Fruit Liver Milk Soya flour Vegetables	Anaemia Appetite loss Dry skin Fatigue Nausea Muscle pain Raised cholesterol levels
C (ascorbic acid)	Citrus fruit Raw cabbage Strawberries Tomatoes	Bleeding gums Poor healing of wounds Scurvy
D (calciferol)	Cod liver oil Fish oil	Rickets (bone deformities)

Vitamin	Food sources (examples)	Deficiency results in
E (tocopherol)	Eggs Meat Milk Liver Vegetables Wheatgerm oil Wholegrain cereals	Anaemia Fluid retention
K	Green leafy vegetables Pork liver	Deficiency is rare

Note! Vitamins are divided into fat-soluble vitamins (A, D, E and K) and water-soluble vitamins (all the B vitamins and vitamin C). Fat-soluble vitamins are stored in the body and do not need to be eaten every day. Water-soluble vitamins dissolve in water and are excreted by the body if we eat too much of them. As they are not stored in the body they must be eaten every day.

Eating too much of any one vitamin can be dangerous and it is unwise to take vitamin supplements without first consulting your doctor. When certain vitamins are taken in excess of the body's requirements they act as toxins and are particularly harmful. For example, too much niacin can cause liver damage in some people.

Mineral	Food sources (examples)	Deficiency results in
Calcium	Beans Cheese Fish (eaten with bones) Milk	Rickets Stunted growth Weak bones in adults
Chloride	Salt	Appetite loss Mental apathy Muscle cramps
Magnesium	Beans Green leafy vegetables Milk Nuts	Anxiety Depression Muscle tremors
Phosphorus	Beans Cheese Fish Milk Nuts White meat Whole grains	Deficiency is rare
Potassium	Cereals Fruit (especially bananas) Salt Vegetables (especially potatoes)	Deficiency is rare

Mineral	Food sources (examples)	Deficiency results in
Sodium	Bacon Kippers Salt Yeast extract	Apathy Appetite loss Fainting Muscular cramps
Sulphur	Beans Eggs Fish Meat	Deficiency is rare

In addition to the major minerals listed here, our bodies also need certain minerals in very minute amounts. These "trace minerals" – chromium, copper, fluoride, iodine, iron, manganese, molybdenum, selenium and zinc – come from a wide variety of foods.

It is common to find mineral supplements in health food shops and chemists. However, as for vitamins, it is advisable to consult your doctor before taking supplements as too much of any one mineral can be dangerous. For example, excess calcium may cause diarrhoea, kidney damage and vomiting; excess fluoride causes discolouration of the teeth; and too much iodine prevents the thyroid gland from functioning properly.

Conversion table

Converting imperial to metric

1 ounce (oz)	= 28.349 grams (g)
1 pound (lb)	= 453.6 grams (g)
	= 0.4536 kilograms (kg)
1 stone (st)	= 6.350 kilograms (kg)
1 fluid ounce (fl oz)	= 28.413 millilitres (ml)
1 pint (pt)	= 568 millilitres (ml)
	= 0.568 litre (l)

to convert ounces to grams x 28.349

to convert pounds to kilograms x 0.454

to convert stones to kilograms x 6.350

to convert fluid ounces to millilitres x 28.413

to convert pints to litres x 0.568

Conversion table

Converting metric to imperial

1 gram (g)	= 0.0353 ounces (oz)
1 kilogram (kg)	= 2.205 pounds (lb)
	= 0.157 stone (st)
1 millilitre (ml)	= 0.0352 fluid ounces (fl oz)
1 litre (l)	= 1.76 pints (pt)

to convert grams to ounces x 0.035

to convert kilograms to pounds x 2.205

to convert kilograms to stones x 0.157

to convert millilitres to fluid ounces x 0.035

to convert litres to pints x 1.760

Abbreviations used in this book

Energy
kcal = kilocalorie

Weight
g = gram
kg = kilogram
oz = ounce
lb = pound
st = stone

Volume
ml = millilitre
fl oz = fluid ounce
pt = pint

Length
ft = feet
m = metres
in = inches

Other figures
Tr = trace (less than 0.1 g)
N = information not available
tsp = teaspoon
tbsp = tablespoon

kcal/100 g = the number of kilocalories per 100 grams of food.
kcal/100 ml = the number of kilocalories per 100 millilitres of liquid.
Cal/hour = Calories used per hour.

Calorie Counter – Foods

Warning! Differences between brands

The Calorie and fat contents of products can vary considerably depending on the brand and it is always wise to check food labels carefully. For example, 100 grams of Crosse & Blackwell baked beans contains 75 Calories compared with Holland & Barrett's variety of the same product, which contains only 47 Calories. The majority of the figures given in the Calorie Counter section of this book are average figures and should be used as a guide only. Some brand-name products have also been included to illustrate the differences between brands.

Product	Calories*	Fat*
Beans, baked, canned in tomato sauce	84	0.6
Beans, baked, canned in tomato sauce (Crosse & Blackwell)	75	0.5
Beans, baked, canned in tomato sauce (Heinz)	75	0.2
Beans, baked, canned in tomato sauce (Holland & Barrett)	47	0.2

* Figures given for 100 grams

Food	CALORIES	FAT
Anchovies, canned in oil	280	19.9
Apple chutney	201	0.2
Apple juice, unsweetened	38	0.1
Apples, cooking, raw, peeled	35	0.1
Apples, cooking, stewed	33	0.1
Apples, cooking, stewed with sugar	74	0.1
Apples, eating, raw	47	0.1
Apricots, canned in juice	34	0.1
Apricots, canned in syrup	63	0.1
Apricots, canned in syrup (Del Monte)	72	0.1
Apricots, raw	31	0.1
Apricots, ready-to-eat	158	0.6
Asparagus, boiled	26	0.8
Aubergine, fried in corn oil	302	31.9
Avocado	190	19.5
Bacon, collar joint, boiled	325	27.0

Calories measured in kcal per 100g/100ml *Fat measured as a % of 100g/100ml*

Food	CALORIES	FAT
Bacon, collar joint, boiled, lean only	191	9.7
Bacon, cooked	692	72.8
Bacon, gammon joint, boiled	269	18.9
Bacon, gammon joint, boiled, lean only	167	5.5
Bacon, gammon rasher, grilled	228	12.2
Bacon, gammon rasher, grilled, lean only	172	5.2
Bacon, rasher, fried, back	465	40.6
Bacon, rasher, fried, lean only	332	22.3
Bacon, rasher, fried, middle	477	42.3
Bacon, rasher, fried, streaky	96	44.8
Bacon, rasher, grilled, back	405	33.8
Bacon, rasher, grilled, lean only	292	18.9
Bacon, rasher, grilled, middle	416	35.1
Bacon, rasher, grilled, streaky	422	36.0

Calories measured in kcal per 100g/100ml *Fat measured as a % of 100g/100ml*

Food	CALORIES	FAT
Baking powder	163	Tr
Bananas	95	0.3
Bananas, dried (Holland & Barrett)	210	Tr
Beans, aduki, dried, boiled	123	0.2
Beans, baked, in tomato sauce	84	0.6
Beans, baked, in tomato sauce (Crosse & Blackwell)	75	0.5
Beans, baked, in tomato sauce (Heinz)	75	0.2
Beans, baked, in tomato sauce (Holland & Barrett)	47	0.2
Beans, baked, in tomato sauce, no added sugar (Heinz)	56	0.2
Beans, baked, in tomato sauce, reduced sugar, reduced salt	73	0.6

Calories measured in kcal per 100g/100ml *Fat measured as a % of 100g/100ml*

Food	CALORIES	FAT
Beans, baked, with bacon (Heinz)	91	1.7
Beans, baked, with burgerbites (Heinz)	103	2.8
Beans, baked, with hotdogs (Heinz)	110	5.0
Beans, baked, with low-fat pork sausages (Crosse & Blackwell)	91.0	2.7
Beans, baked, with mini sausages (Heinz)	117	4.5
Beans, baked, with pepperoni (Heinz)	93.0	1.9
Beans, baked, with pork sausages (Heinz)	110	4.3
Beans, baked, with vegetable sausages (Crosse & Blackwell)	120	5.3
Beans, barbecue (Heinz)	90.0	0.5
Beans, barlotti (Napolina)	70	0.3

Calories measured in kcal per 100g/100ml *Fat measured as a % of 100g/100ml*

Food	CALORIES	FAT
Beans, blackeye, dried, boiled	116	0.7
Beans, broad, frozen, boiled	81	0.6
Beans, butter, canned	77	0.5
Beans, cannelini (Batchelors)	100	0.7
Beans, flageolet (Batchelors)	98	0.7
Beans, French/green, frozen, boiled	25	0.1
Beans, mung, dried, boiled	91	0.4
Beans, red kidney, canned	100	0.6
Beans, red kidney, dried, boiled	103	0.5
Beans, runner, boiled	18	0.5
Beans, soya, dried, boiled	141	7.3
Beansprouts, mung, raw	31	0.5
Beansprouts, mung, stir-fried in blended oil	72	6.1
Beef, brisket, boiled	326	23.9
Beef, cooked	613	62.8

Calories measured in kcal per 100g/100ml *Fat measured as a % of 100g/100ml*

Food	CALORIES	FAT
Beef, forerib, roast	349	28.8
Beef, forerib, roast, lean only	225	12.6
Beef, minced, stewed	229	15.2
Beef, rump steak, fried	246	14.6
Beef, rump steak, fried, lean only	190	7.4
Beef, rump steak, grilled	218	12.1
Beef, rump steak, grilled, lean only	168	6.0
Beef, silverside, salted, boiled	242	14.2
Beef, silverside, salted, boiled, lean only	173	4.9
Beef, sirloin, roast	284	21.1
Beef, sirloin, roast, lean only	192	9.1
Beef, stewed steak	223	11.0
Beef, topside, roast	214	12.0
Beef, topside, roast, lean only	156	4.4
Beefburgers, frozen fried	264	17.3

Calories measured in kcal per 100g/100ml *Fat measured as a % of 100g/100ml*

Food	CALORIES	FAT
Beef chow mein	136	6.0
Beef curry	137	6.6
Beef kheema	413	37.7
Beef koftas	353	27.6
Beef steak pudding	224	12.3
Beef steak, stewed, canned	176	12.5
Beef stew	120	7.2
Beetroot, boiled	46	0.1
Beetroot, pickled	28	0.2
Biscuits, Abbey Crunch (McVitie's)	479	18.0
Biscuits, Animal (Cadbury)	493	20.6
Biscuits, bourbons (Jacob's)	464	21.7
Biscuits, chocolate	524	27.6
Biscuits, chocolate chip cookies (Cadbury)	484	20.6
Biscuits, digestive, chocolate	493	24.1

Calories measured in kcal per 100g/100ml *Fat measured as a % of 100g/100ml*

Food	CALORIES	FAT
Biscuits, digestive, chocolate (Holland & Barrett)	487	23.6
Biscuits, digestive, plain	471	20.9
Biscuits, fig rolls (Jacob's)	363	7.1
Biscuits, filled wafers	535	29.9
Biscuits, Fruit Club (Jacob's)	496	25.0
Biscuits, gingernut	456	15.2
Biscuits, Penguin (McVitie's)	447	16.0
Biscuits, Rich Tea (McVitie's)	470	15.7
Biscuits, Rich Water (Jacob's)	436	13.3
Biscuits, Shortcake (Jacob's)	464	21.2
Black pudding, fried	305	21.9
Blackberries, raw	25	0.2
Blackberries, stewed	21	0.2
Blackberries, stewed with sugar	56	0.2
Blackcurrants, canned in juice	31	Tr
Blackcurrants, canned in syrup	72	Tr

Calories measured in kcal per 100g/100ml *Fat measured as a % of 100g/100ml*

Food	CALORIES	FAT
Blackcurrants, raw	Tr	26
Blackcurrants, stewed with sugar	58	Tr
Bombay mix	503	32.9
Bran	206	5.5
Brawn	153	11.5
Bread, brown	218	2.0
Bread, brown, toasted	328	12.8
Bread, currant	289	7.6
Bread, currant toasted	323	8.5
Bread, French stick	270	2.7
Bread, granary	235	2.7
Bread, malt	268	2.4
Bread, naan	336	12.5
Bread, oatmeal (Crofters Kitchen)	234	3.9
Bread, pitta, white	265	1.2

Calories measured in kcal per 100g/100ml *Fat measured as a % of 100g/100ml*

Food	CALORIES	FAT
Bread, rye	219	1.7
Bread, white	235	1.9
Bread, white, toasted	265	1.6
Bread, wholemeal	215	2.5
Bread, wholemeal, toasted	252	2.9
Bread pudding	297	9.6
Bread rolls, crusty, brown	255	2.8
Bread rolls, crusty, white	280	2.3
Bread rolls, soft, brown	268	3.8
Bread rolls, soft, white	268	4.2
Bread rolls, wholemeal	241	2.9
Breakfast cereals, All-Bran, (Kellogg's)	270	3.5
Breakfast cereals, Alpen, (Weetabix)	364	6.8
Breakfast cereals, Alpen, no added sugar (Weetabix)	363	7.2
Breakfast cereals, bran flakes	318	1.9

Calories measured in kcal per 100g/100ml *Fat measured as a % of 100g/100ml*

Food	CALORIES	FAT
Breakfast cereals, Bran Flakes (Kellogg's)	320	2.0
Breakfast cereals, Coco Pops (Kellogg's)	380	0.8
Breakfast cereals, Common Sense Oat Bran Flakes (Kellogg's)	360	5.0
Breakfast cereals, corn flakes	360	0.7
Breakfast cereals, Corn Flakes (Kellogg's)	370	0.7
Breakfast cereals, Country Bran (Jordan's)	206	5.5
Breakfast cereals, Country Muesli (Jordan's)	350	5.9
Breakfast cereals, Crunchy Nut Cornflakes (Kellogg's)	390	3.5
Breakfast cereals, Deluxe Muesli (Holland & Barrett)	356	11.1
Breakfast cereals, Frosties (Kellogg's)	380	0.5

Calories measured in kcal per 100g/100ml *Fat measured as a % of 100g/100ml*

Food	CALORIES	FAT
Breakfast cereals, Fruit 'n' Fibre (Kellogg's)	350	6.0
Breakfast cereals, Harvest Crunch (Quaker)	449	16.0
Muesli, Swiss style	363	5.9
Muesli, Swiss style, no added sugar	366	7.8
Breakfast cereals, porridge, made with water	49	1.1
Breakfast cereals, Porridge Oats (Whitworths)	401	8.7
Breakfast cereals, Puffed Wheat (Quaker)	328	1.3
Breakfast cereals, Ready Brek (Weetabix)	359	8.4
Breakfast cereals, Ready Brek, chocolate (Weetabix)	377	9.7
Breakfast cereals, Rice Krispies (Kellogg's)	370	0.9

Calories measured in kcal per 100g/100ml *Fat measured as a % of 100g/100ml*

Food	CALORIES	FAT
Breakfast cereals, Scotts Porridge Oats (Quaker)	366	7.6
Breakfast cereals, Sugar Puffs (Quaker)	387	1.0
Breakfast cereals, Weetabix (Weetabix)	342	2.7
Broccoli, boiled	24	0.8
Brussels sprouts, boiled	35	1.3
Buns, Chelsea	366	13.8
Buns, currant	296	7.5
Buns, hot cross	310	6.8
Butter	737	81.7
Butter-type spreads, dairy/fat	622	73.4
Butter-type spreads, low-fat	390	40.5
Butter-type spreads, Olivio, Reduced Fat Spread (Van den Bergh)	544	60.0
Butter-type spreads, Outline Very Low Fat Spread (Van den Bergh)	222	22.5

Calories measured in kcal per 100g/100ml *Fat measured as a % of 100g/100ml*

Food	CALORIES	FAT
Butter-type spreads, very low-fat	273	25.0
Cabbage, boiled	16	0.4
Cabbage, January King, boiled	18	0.6
Cabbage, white, raw	27	0.2
Cake, Bakewell tart (Mr Kipling)	436	18.5
Cake, banana (California Cake & Cookie Ltd)	328	10.0
Cake, battenburg (Mr Kipling)	380	9.9
Cake, chocolate (Cadbury)	384	14.2
Cake, chocolate (Lyons Bakeries)	467	27.0
Cake, chocolate Swiss roll (Mr Kipling)	328	12.5
Cake, Christmas (Mr Kipling)	360	8.5
Cake, Christmas log (Mr Kipling)	435	19.0

Calories measured in kcal per 100g/100ml *Fat measured as a % of 100g/100ml*

Food	CALORIES	FAT
Cake, Country Fruit Cake (Mr Kipling)	377	15.0
Cake, cream horns	435	35.8
Cake, cupcakes, assorted (Lyons Bakeries)	358	5.5
Cake, custard tarts	277	14.5
Cake, Danish pastries	374	17.6
Cake, doughnuts, jam	336	14.5
Cake, doughnuts, ring	397	21.7
Cake, Eccles	475	26.4
Cake, eclairs, frozen	396	30.6
Cake, gateau	337	16.8
Cake, Greek pastries	322	17.0
Cake, Jaffa Cakes (McVitie's)	367	8.2
Cake, jam tarts	368	13.0
Cake, lemon curd tarts (Lyons Bakeries)	417	17.5
Cake, Madeira	393	16.9

Calories measured in kcal per 100g/100ml *Fat measured as a % of 100g/100ml*

Food	CALORIES	FAT
Cake, mince pies	423	20.4
Cake, mince pies (Holland & Barrett)	318	16.1
Cake, plain fruit	354	12.9
Cake, rich fruit	341	11.0
Cake, rich fruit, iced	356	11.4
Cake, sponge	459	26.3
Cake, sponge, fatless	294	6.1
Cake, sponge, jam filled	302	4.9
Cake, sponge, with butter icing	490	30.6
Cake, Swiss roll, chocolate	337	11.3
Cake, Swiss roll, jam (Mr Kipling)	211	2.3
Cake, Swiss roll, raspberry (Lyons Bakeries)	307	1.7
Cake, Swiss roll, raspberry and vanilla (Lyons Bakeries)	341	8.3

Calories measured in kcal per 100g/100ml *Fat measured as a % of 100g/100ml*

Food	CALORIES	FAT
Cake, wholemeal fruit	363	15.7
Carnation Slender Plan Drink made with whole milk, chocolate flavour	229	8.2
Carnation Slender Plan Drink made with whole milk, coffee flavour	228	7.8
Carnation Slender Plan Drink made with whole milk, raspberry	228	7.8
Carnation Slender Plan Drink made with whole milk, strawberry flavour	228	7.8
Carnation Slender Plan Drink made with whole milk, vanilla flavour	230	7.8
Carrots, canned	20	0.3
Carrots, old, boiled	24	0.4
Carrots, old, raw	35	0.3

Calories measured in kcal per 100g/100ml *Fat measured as a % of 100g/100ml*

Food	CALORIES	FAT
Carrots, young, boiled	22	0.4
Carrots, young, raw	30	0.5
Cauliflower, boiled	28	0.9
Cauliflower cheese	105	6.9
Celery, boiled	8	0.3
Celery, raw	7	0.2
Cheese, Boursin au Concombreau (Van den Bergh)	233	21
Cheese, Brie	319	26.9
Cheese, Camembert	297	23.7
Cheese, Cheddar	412	34.4
Cheese, Cheddar, reduced fat	261	15.0
Cheese, Cheddar, slices (Kraft)	325	26.0
Cheese, Cheddar, vegetarian	425	35.7
Cheese, cottage, plain	98	3.9
Cheese, cottage, plain (Eden Vale)	85	1.5
Cheese, cottage, reduced fat	78	1.4

Calories measured in kcal per 100g/100ml *Fat measured as a % of 100g/100ml*

Food	CALORIES	FAT
Cheese, cottage, with additions	95	3.8
Cheese, cottage, with onion and chives (Eden Vale)	105	4.0
Cheese, cream	439	47.4
Cheese, Danish blue	347	29.6
Cheese, Edam	333	25.4
Cheese, feta	250	20.2
Cheese, Gouda	375	31.0
Cheese, hard	405	34.0
Cheese, Lymeswold	425	40.3
Cheese, Parmesan	452	32.7
Cheese, processed, plain	330	27.0
Cheese, soft, full-fat	313	31.0
Cheese, soft, full-fat, Philadelphia (Kraft)	310	30.0
Cheese, soft, medium-fat	179	14.5
Cheese, soft, medium-fat, Philadelphia (Kraft)	185	15.0

Calories measured in kcal per 100g/100ml *Fat measured as a % of 100g/100ml*

Food	CALORIES	FAT
Cheese, soft, medium-fat, Philadelphia with pineapple (Kraft)	185	11.5
Cheese, soft, medium-fat, Philadelphia with salmon (Kraft)	187	15.0
Cheesecake, blackcurrant (Eden Vale)	262	11.7
Cheesecake, blackcurrant (Heinz)	160	4.1
Cheesecake, blackcurrant (McVitie's)	295	17.0
Cheesecake, frozen	242	10.6
Cheesecake, raspberry (Young's)	298	17.1
Cheesecake, strawberry (Heinz)	160	4.0
Cheesecake, strawberry (McVitie's)	385	22.0

Calories measured in kcal per 100g/100ml *Fat measured as a % of 100g/100ml*

Food	CALORIES	FAT
Cheese spread, plain	276	22.8
Cheese spread, Dairylea (Kraft)	281	23.2
Cheese, Stilton, blue	411	35.5
Cheese, white	376	31.3
Cherries, black, canned in syrup (Libby)	73	Tr
Cherries, canned in syrup	71	Tr
Cherries, cocktail (Burgess)	247	0
Cherries, glacé	251	Tr
Cherries, raw	48	0.1
Chick peas, canned	115	2.9
Chick peas, dried, boiled	121	2.1
Chicken, boiled, dark meat	204	9.9
Chicken, boiled, light meat	163	4.9
Chicken, boiled, meat only	183	7.3
Chicken, breaded, fried in vegetable oil	242	12.7

Calories measured in kcal per 100g/100ml *Fat measured as a % of 100g/100ml*

Food	CALORIES	FAT
Chicken, roast, dark meat	155	6.9
Chicken, roast, leg quarter, meat only, weighed with bone	92	3.4
Chicken, roast, light meat	142	4.0
Chicken, roast, meat and skin	216	14.0
Chicken, roast, meat only	148	5.4
Chicken, roast, wing quarter, meat only, weighed with bone	74	2.7
Chicken curry	205	17.0
Chicory, raw	11	0.6
Chilli con carne	151	8.5
Chilli powder	N	16.8
Chips, fine cut, frozen, fried in blended oil	364	21.3
Chips, fine cut, frozen, fried in corn oil	364	21.3

Calories measured in kcal per 100g/100ml *Fat measured as a % of 100g/100ml*

Food	CALORIES	FAT
Chips, fine cut, frozen, fried in dripping	364	21.3
Chips, home-made, fried in blended oil	189	6.7
Chips, home-made, fried in corn oil	189	6.7
Chips, home-made, fried in dripping	189	6.7
Chips, microwave, Crinkle Microchips (McCain)	187	8.2
Chips, oven, frozen, baked	162	4.2
Chips, oven, Crinkle Oven Chips (McCain)	157	4.7
Chips, straight cut, frozen, fried in blended oil	273	13.5
Chips, straight cut, frozen, fried in corn oil	273	13.5
Chips, straight cut, frozen, fried in dripping	273	13.5

Calories measured in kcal per 100g/100ml *Fat measured as a % of 100g/100ml*

Food	CALORIES	FAT
Chocolate, Aero Minibars (Nestlé)	518	28.8
Chocolate, Aero, Mint (Nestlé)	526	28.8
Chocolate, Aero, Orange (Nestlé)	526	28.8
Chocolate, After Eight Mints (Nestlé)	419	13.3
Chocolate, Animal Bar (Nestlé)	512	26.5
Chocolate, Bounty, dark (Mars)	482	27.0
Chocolate, Bounty, milk (Mars)	486	27.0
Chocolate, Bournville (Cadbury)	496	27.0
Chocolate, Bournville Fruit and Nut (Cadbury)	495	23.0
Chocolate, Buttons (Cadbury)	526	30.0

Calories measured in kcal per 100g/100ml *Fat measured as a % of 100g/100ml*

Food	CALORIES	FAT
Chocolate, Chunky Aero (Nestlé)	530	31.1
Chocolate, Coffee Matchmakers (Nestlé)	474	21.4
Chocolate, Crunchie (Cadbury)	490	18.8
Chocolate, Curly Wurly (Cadbury)	425	17.0
Chocolates, filled	464	18.0
Chocolate, Flake (Cadbury)	530	30.7
Chocolate, Double Decker (Cadbury)	465	18.1
Chocolate, Fruit and Nut (Cadbury)	474	24.0
Chocolate, Galaxy (Mars)	488	25.0
Chocolate, Galaxy Caramel (Mars)	488	25.1
Chocolate, Galaxy Double Nut and Raisin (Mars)	533	30.7

Calories measured in kcal per 100g/100ml *Fat measured as a % of 100g/100ml*

Food	CALORIES	FAT
Chocolate, Galaxy Hazlenut (Mars)	571	38.5
Chocolate, Galaxy Minstrels (Mars)	490	19.5
Chocolate, Galaxy Ripple (Mars)	531	29.5
Chocolate, Kit Kat (Nestlé)	502	26.0
Chocolate, Maltesers (Mars)	495	24.0
Chocolate, Mars Bar (Mars)	453	18.0
Chocolate, Matchmakers, Mint (Nestlé)	477	20.2
Chocolate, Matchmakers, Orange (Nestlé)	476	20.2
Chocolate, milk	529	30.3
Chocolate, milk (Cadbury)	526	30.0
Chocolate, milk (Nestlé)	520	29.5
Chocolate, Milk Tray (Cadbury)	481	23.4

Calories measured in kcal per 100g/100ml *Fat measured as a % of 100g/100ml*

Food	CALORIES	FAT
Chocolate, Milky Way (Mars)	455	16.7
Chocolate, nut spread	549	33.0
Chocolate, peanut M & Ms (Mars)	513	27.0
Chocolate, plain	525	29.2
Chocolate, Raisin & Biscuit Yorkie (Nestlé)	481	23.8
Chocolate, Rolo (Nestlé)	473	20.8
Chocolate, Roses (Cadbury)	481	23.7
Chocolate, Smarties (Nestlé)	459	17.0
Chocolate, Snickers (Mars)	510	26.4
Chocolate, Toffee Crisp (Nestlé)	494	25.5
Chocolate, Topic (Mars)	497	27.6
Chocolate, Twirl (Cadbury)	526	30.2
Chocolate, Twix (Mars)	495	24.2
Chocolate, white	529	30.9

Calories measured in kcal per 100g/100ml *Fat measured as a % of 100g/100ml*

Food	CALORIES	FAT
Chocolate, white, Milky Bar (Nestlé)	549	32.5
Chocolate, white, Milky Bar Buttons (Nestlé)	549	32.5
Chocolate, Wholenut (Cadbury)	520	29.3
Chocolate, Wildlife (Cadbury)	521	30.0
Chocolate, Yorkie (Nestlé)	526	29.5
Chocolate, Yorkie, Peanut (Nestlé)	526	29.5
Christmas pudding	329	11.8
Chutney, apple	201	0.2
Chutney, apricot	141	0.1
Chutney, curried fruit (Sharwood)	129	0.4
Chutney, mango	285	10.9
Chutney, peach (Sharwood)	163	0.1
Chutney, tomato	162	0.4

Calories measured in kcal per 100g/100ml *Fat measured as a % of 100g/100ml*

Food	CALORIES	FAT
Clementines	37	0.1
Cockles, boiled	48	0.3
Cocoa powder, made with whole milk	76	4.2
Cocoa powder, made with semi-skimmed milk	57	1.9
Cod, dried, salted, boiled	138	0.9
Cod fillets, baked	96	1.2
Cod fillets, poached	94	1.1
Cod steaks, Chip Shop Jumbo Cod Steaks (Ross)	179	10.0
Cod steaks, frozen, grilled	95	1.3
Cod steaks in batter, fried in blended oil	199	10.3
Cod steaks in batter, fried in dripping	199	10.3
Coffee and chicory essence	218	0.2
Coffee, infusion	2	Tr

Calories measured in kcal per 100g/100ml *Fat measured as a % of 100g/100ml*

Food	CALORIES	FAT
Coffee, instant	100	0
Coffee, instant, cappuccino (Nescafé)	385	14.0
Coffee, instant, cappuccino, unsweetened (Nescafé)	393	14.0
Coffee, instant, decaf (Nescafé)	107	Tr
Coffee, instant, standard (Nescafé)	94	Tr
Cola	39	0
Cola (Pepsi)	44	0
Cola diet (Pepsi)	0.25	0
Coleslaw (Heinz)	133	10.0
Coleslaw (St Ivel)	95	7.4
Cooking fat, compound	894	99.3
Corned beef	217	12.1
Cornflour	354	0.7
Cornish pastie	332	20.4

Calories measured in kcal per 100g/100ml *Fat measured as a % of 100g/100ml*

Food	CALORIES	FAT
Courgette, boiled	19	0.4
Courgette, fried in corn oil	63	4.8
Crab, boiled	127	5.2
Crab, canned	81	0.9
Crackers, cream	440	16.3
Crackers, wholemeal	413	11.3
Cranberry jelly (Baxters)	255	Tr
Cream, clotted	586	63.5
Cream, double	449	48.0
Cream, half	148	13.3
Cream, single	198	19.1
Cream, soured	205	19.9
Cream, sterilised, canned	239	23.9
Cream, UHT, canned spray	309	32.0
Cream, whipping	373	39.3
Cream alternatives, Delight Double Cream (Van den Bergh)	244	24.1

Calories measured in kcal per 100g/100ml *Fat measured as a % of 100g/100ml*

Food	CALORIES	FAT
Cream alternatives, Delight Whipping Cream (Van den Bergh)	196	18.4
Cream alternatives, Dessert Top (Nestlé)	292	30.0
Cream alternatives, Emlea, Double (Van den Bergh)	412	44.0
Cream alternatives, Emlea, Single (Van den Bergh)	184	18.0
Cream alternatives, Emlea, Whipping (Van den Bergh)	320	32.0
Cream alternatives, Flora, double (Van den Bergh)	70	7.4
Cream alternatives, Flora, single (Van den Bergh)	31	2.9
Cream alternatives, Tip Top (Nestlé)	113	6.2
Crème caramel	109	2.2
Crispbread, rye	321	2.1

Calories measured in kcal per 100g/100ml *Fat measured as a % of 100g/100ml*

Food	CALORIES	FAT
Crisps	546	37.6
Crisps, low-fat	456	21.5
Croissants	360	20.3
Crumpets, toasted	199	1.0
Cucumber, raw	10	0.1
Curly kale, boiled	24	1.1
Currants	267	0.4
Custard, canned	95	3.0
Custard, canned, low-fat (Ambrosia)	75	1.4
Custard, made with skimmed milk	79	0.1
Custard, made with whole milk	117	4.5
Custard, powder	354	0.7
Custard, ready to serve (Bird's)	100	3.0
Damsons, raw	34	Tr
Damsons, stewed with sugar	74	Tr

Calories measured in kcal per 100g/100ml *Fat measured as a % of 100g/100ml*

Food	CALORIES	FAT
Dandelion and Burdock (Barr)	28	Tr
Dates, raw	107	0.1
Dogfish in batter, fried in dripping	265	18.8
Dogfish in batter, fried in blended oil	265	18.8
Drinking chocolate powder, made with semi-skimmed milk	71	1.9
Drinking chocolate powder, made with whole milk	90	4.1
Dripping, beef	891	99.0
Duck, roast, meat, fat and skin	339	29.0
Duck, roast, meat only	189	9.7
Dumplings	208	11.7
Egg white, chicken, raw	36	Tr
Egg yolk, chicken, raw	339	30.5
Eggs, chicken, boiled	147	10.8

Calories measured in kcal per 100g/100ml *Fat measured as a % of 100g/100ml*

Food	CALORIES	FAT
Eggs, chicken, fried in vegetable oil	179	13.9
Eggs, chicken, poached	147	10.8
Eggs, chicken, scrambled, with milk	247	22.6
Eggs, chicken, whole, raw	147	10.8
Eggs, duck, whole, raw	163	11.8
Eggs, Scotch	251	17.1
Faggots	268	18.5
Fennel, Florence, boiled	11	0.2
Fennel, Florence, raw	12	0.2
Figs, dried	227	1.6
Figs, ready-to-eat	209	1.5
Fish cakes, Chip Shop Fish Cakes (Ross)	231	12.6
Fish cakes, fried	188	10.5
Fish fingers, Chip Shop Jumbo Cod Fish Fingers (Ross)	231	15.1

Calories measured in kcal per 100g/100ml *Fat measured as a % of 100g/100ml*

Food	CALORIES	FAT
Fish fingers, cod (Ross)	182	8.7
Fish fingers, fried in blended oil	233	12.7
Fish fingers, fried in lard	233	12.7
Fish fingers, grilled	214	9.0
Fish paste	169	10.4
Fish pie	105	3.0
Frankfurters	274	25.0
Fromage frais, fruit	131	5.8
Fromage frais, orange sorbet (St Ivel)	51	0.1
Fromage frais, peach (Ski)	124	4.8
Fromage frais, plain	113	7.1
Fromage frais, raspberry (St Ivel)	47	0.1
Fromage frais, strawberry (St Ivel)	50	0.1
Fromage frais, strawberry (Ski)	123	4.8

Calories measured in kcal per 100g/100ml *Fat measured as a % of 100g/100ml*

Food	CALORIES	FAT
Fromage frais, very low-fat	58	0.2
Fruit, mixed, dried	268	0.4
Fruit cocktail, canned in juice	29	Tr
Fruit cocktail, canned in syrup	57	Tr
Fruit, crumble, fruit	198	6.9
Fruit, crumble, fruit, wholemeal	193	7.1
Fruit pie, apple (Lyons Bakeries)	370	15.1
Fruit pie, apple (McVitie's)	236	10.0
Fruit pie, blackcurrant, with pastry top and bottom	262	13.3
Fruit pie, individual	369	15.5
Fruit pie, one crust	186	7.9
Fruit pie, pastry top and bottom	260	13.3
Fruit pie, wholemeal, one crust	183	8.1

Calories measured in kcal per 100g/100ml *Fat measured as a % of 100g/100ml*

Food	CALORIES	FAT
Fruit pie, wholemeal, pastry	251	13.6
Gelatin	338	0
Ghee, butter	898	99.8
Ghee, palm	897	99.7
Ghee, vegetable	898	99.8
Gherkins, pickled	14	0.1
Ginger ale, American (Schweppes)	22	N
Ginger ale, dry (Schweppes)	16	N
Ginger ale, Slimline American (Schweppes)	0.7	N
Ginger beer (Schweppes)	34.7	N
Goose, roast, meat only	319	22.4
Gooseberries, cooking, raw	19	0.4
Gooseberries, dessert, canned in syrup	73	0.2
Gooseberries, stewed	16	0.3
Gooseberries, stewed with sugar	54	0.3

Calories measured in kcal per 100g/100ml *Fat measured as a % of 100g/100ml*

Food	CALORIES	FAT
Gourd, karela, raw	11	0.2
Grapefruit, canned in juice	30	Tr
Grapefruit, canned in syrup	60	Tr
Grapefruit, raw	30	0.1
Grapes	60	0.1
Gravy granules, average, made up with water	33	2.4
Gravy granules, chicken, made up (RHM Foods)	37	2.7
Gravy granules, onion, made up (RHM Foods)	36	2.5
Grouse, roast, meat only	173	5.3
Guava, canned in syrup	60	Tr
Guava, raw	26	0.5
Haddock, smoked, steamed	101	0.9
Haddock, steamed	98	0.8
Haddock in crumbs, fried in blended oil	174	8.3

Calories measured in kcal per 100g/100ml *Fat measured as a % of 100g/100ml*

Food	CALORIES	FAT
Haddock in crumbs, fried in dripping	174	8.3
Haggis, boiled	310	21.7
Halibut, steamed	131	4.0
Ham, canned	120	5.1
Ham and pork, chopped, canned	275	23.6
Hamburger buns	264	5.0
Hare, stewed, meat only	192	8.0
Heart, ox, stewed	179	5.9
Heart, sheep, roast	237	14.7
Herbs and spices, cinnamon, ground	N	3.2
Herbs and spices, curry powder	233	10.8
Herbs and spices, garam masala	379	15.1
Herbs and spices, garlic, raw	98	0.6

Calories measured in kcal per 100g/100ml *Fat measured as a % of 100g/100ml*

Food	CALORIES	FAT
Herbs and spices, mint, fresh	43	0.7
Herbs and spices, nutmeg, ground	N	36.3
Herbs and spices, paprika	289	13.0
Herbs and spices, parsley, fresh	34	1.3
Herbs and spices, pepper, black	N	3.3
Herbs and spices, pepper, white	N	2.1
Herbs and spices, rosemary, dried	331	15.2
Herbs and spices, sage, dried, ground	315	12.7
Herbs and spices, thyme, dried, ground	276	7.4
Herring, fried	234	15.1
Herring, grilled	199	13.0
Honey	288	0

Calories measured in kcal per 100g/100ml *Fat measured as a % of 100g/100ml*

Food	CALORIES	FAT
Honeycomb	281	4.6
Hummus	187	12.6
Ice cream, arctic roll	200	6.6
Ice cream, choc ice	277	17.5
Ice cream, chocolate (Fiesta)	186	10.5
Ice cream, chocolate (Lyons Maid)	90	4.1
Ice cream, chocolate nut sundae	278	15.3
Ice cream, Cornish (Lyons Maid)	91	4.3
Ice cream, dairy, flavoured	179	8.0
Ice cream, dairy, vanilla	194	9.8
Ice cream, frozen dessert	226	14.1
Ice cream, lemon sorbet	131	Tr
Ice cream, Neopolitan (Fiesta)	174	9.5
Ice cream, Neopolitan (Lyons Maid)	88	4.1

Calories measured in kcal per 100g/100ml *Fat measured as a % of 100g/100ml*

Food	CALORIES	FAT
Ice cream, non-dairy, flavoured	166	7.4
Ice cream, non-dairy, vanilla	178	8.7
Ice cream, raspberry ripple (Fiesta)	193	10.0
Ice cream, raspberry ripple (Lyons Maid)	115	4.0
Ice cream, strawberry (Heinz)	133	5.6
Ice cream, strawberry (Fiesta)	177	10.5
Ice cream, strawberry (Lyons Maid)	84	3.8
Ice cream, vanilla (Heinz)	142	5.5
Ice cream, vanilla (Fiesta)	154	7.7
Ice cream, vanilla (Lyons Maid)	87	4.5
Ice cream, vanilla, soft scoop (Fiesta)	162	8.5
Instant dessert, made with skimmed milk	97	3.2

Calories measured in kcal per 100g/100ml *Fat measured as a % of 100g/100ml*

Food	CALORIES	FAT
Instant dessert, made with whole milk	125	6.3
Irish stew	123	7.6
Jam, apricot, reduced sugar (Heinz)	126	0
Jam, blackcurrant (Baxters)	210	Tr
Jam, blackcurrant, reduced sugar (Heinz)	126	0
Jam, forest fruits, reduced sugar (Heinz)	127	0.1
Jam, fruit with edible seeds	261	0
Jam, morello cherry, reduced sugar (Heinz)	127	0
Jam, raspberry, reduced sugar (Heinz)	125	0.3
Jam, reduced sugar	123	0.1
Jam, strawberry, reduced sugar (Heinz)	126	0.1
Jam, stone fruit	261	0

Calories measured in kcal per 100g/100ml *Fat measured as a % of 100g/100ml*

Food	CALORIES	FAT
Jelly	61	0
Juice, apple (Britvic 55)	46	Tr
Juice, apple (Del Monte)	43	Tr
Juice, apple, diluted (Robinsons)	88	Tr
Juice, apple, low-calorie drink, bottled (Tango)	4	Tr
Juice, apple, unsweetened	38	0.1
Juice, apple and blackcurrant, diluted (Robinsons)	48	Tr
Juice, apple and raspberry, diluted (Robinsons)	48.	Tr
Juice, apple and strawberry, diluted (Robinsons)	88	Tr
Juice, blackcurrant, undiluted (Ribena)	285	N
Juice, cherry (Robinsons)	45	Tr
Juice, grape, unsweetened	46	0.1

Calories measured in kcal per 100g/100ml *Fat measured as a % of 100g/100ml*

Food	CALORIES	FAT
Juice, grapefruit, unsweetened	33	0.1
Juice, lemon	7	Tr
Juice, lemon drink, diluted (Quosh)	20	N
Juice, lemon drink, low-calorie (Tango)	4	Tr
Juice, lemon drink, no added sugar, diluted (Robinsons)	9.8	Tr
Juice, lemonade, bottled	21	0
Juice, lemonade, bottled (R Whites)	20	Tr
Juice, lemonade, bottled, low-calorie (R Whites)	0.5	N
Juice, lime juice cordial, undiluted	112	0
Juice, lime cordial, diluted (Britvic)	17	Tr
Juice, Lucozade light (SmithKline Beecham)	37	0

Calories measured in kcal per 100g/100ml *Fat measured as a % of 100g/100ml*

Food	CALORIES	FAT
Juice, Lucozade Orange Sport (SmithKline Beecham)	28	0
Juice, orange, undiluted	107	0
Juice, orange, unsweetened	36	0.1
Juice, orange and pineapple (Del Monte)	42	Tr
Juice, orange and pineapple (Tango)	46	Tr
Juice, orange and pineapple, low-calorie (Tango)	3	Tr
Juice, orange and pineapple, sparkling (Tango)	44	N
Juice, pineapple, unsweetened	41	0.1
Juice, Ribena, undiluted	228	0
Juice, tomato	14	Tr
Kedgeree	166	7.9
Kidney, lamb, fried	155	6.3
Kidney, ox, stewed	172	7.7
Kidney, pig, stewed	153	6.1

Calories measured in kcal per 100g/100ml *Fat measured as a % of 100g/100ml*

Food	CALORIES	FAT
Kipper, baked	205	11.4
Kiwi fruit	49	0.5
Lamb, chops, grilled	355	29.0
Lamb, chops, grilled, loin, lean only	222	12.3
Lamb, cooked	616	63.4
Lamb, cutlets, grilled	370	30.9
Lamb, cutlets, grilled, lean only	222	12.3
Lamb, breast, roast	410	37.1
Lamb, breast, roast, lean only	252	16.6
Lamb, leg, roast	266	17.9
Lamb, leg, roast, lean only	91	8.1
Lamb, shoulder, roast	316	26.3
Lamb, shoulder, roast, lean only	196	11.2
Lamb, scrag and neck, stewed	292	21.1

Calories measured in kcal per 100g/100ml *Fat measured as a % of 100g/100ml*

Food	CALORIES	FAT
Lamb, scrag and neck, stewed, lean only	253	15.7
Lamb kheema	328	29.1
Lard	891	99.0
Lasagne, frozen, cooked	102	3.8
Leeks, boiled	21	0.7
Lemon curd	283	5.1
Lemon meringue pie	319	14.4
Lemon sole, steamed	91	0.9
Lemon sole in crumbs, fried	216	13.0
Lemons	19	0.3
Lentils, green and brown, whole, dried, boiled	105	0.7
Lentils, red, split, dried, boiled	100	0.4
Lettuce, butterhead, raw	12	0.6
Lettuce, iceberg	13	0.3
Lettuce, raw	14	0.5

Calories measured in kcal per 100g/100ml *Fat measured as a % of 100g/100ml*

Food	CALORIES	FAT
Liver, calf, fried	254	13.2
Liver, chicken, fried	194	10.9
Liver, lamb, fried	232	14.0
Liver, ox, stewed	198	9.5
Liver, pig, stewed	189	8.1
Liver sausage	310	26.9
Lobster, boiled	119	3.4
Luncheon meat, canned	313	26.9
Lychees, canned in syrup	68	Tr
Lychees, raw	58	0.1
Macaroni, boiled	86	0.5
Macaroni, creamed (Ambrosia)	90	1.7
Macaroni cheese	178	10.8
Mackerel, fried	188	11.3
Mackerel, smoked	354	30.9
Mandarin oranges, canned in juice	32	Tr

Calories measured in kcal per 100g/100ml *Fat measured as a % of 100g/100ml*

Food	CALORIES	FAT
Mandarin oranges, canned in syrup	52	Tr
Mangoes, canned in syrup	77	Tr
Mangoes, ripe, raw	57	0.2
Margarine	739	81.6
Margarine, hard, animal and vegetable fat	739	81.6
Margarine, hard, vegetable fat	739	81.6
Margarine, polyunsaturated	739	81.6
Margarine, soft, animal and vegetable fat	739	81.6
Margarine, soft, vegetable fat	739	81.6
Margarine, Stork (Van den Bergh)	732	81.1
Marmalade	261	0
Marmalade, orange (Baxters)	210	0
Marmalade, orange, reduced sugar (Heinz)	127	0

Calories measured in kcal per 100g/100ml *Fat measured as a % of 100g/100ml*

Food	CALORIES	FAT
Marrow, boiled	9	0.2
Marzipan	404	14.4
Mayonnaise	691	75.6
Mayonnaise, Real Mayonnaise (Hellmans)	720	79.1
Mayonnaise, reduced calorie (Heinz)	275	26.5
Meatballs in gravy (Campbell's)	104	7.0
Meatballs in tomato sauce (Campbell's)	113	6.9
Meat, curried	162	10.5
Meat hot pot	114	4.5
Meat paste	173	11.2
Meat pie, beef and kidney (Tyne Brand)	153	8.0
Meat pie, steak and kidney	323	21.2
Meat pie, steak and kidney (Ross)	271	16.9

Calories measured in kcal per 100g/100ml *Fat measured as a % of 100g/100ml*

Food	CALORIES	FAT
Melon, cantaloupe	19	0.1
Melon, galia	24	0.1
Melon, honeydew	28	0.1
Melon, watermelon	31	0.3
Meringue	379	Tr
Meringue, with cream	376	23.6
Milk pudding, made with skimmed milk	93	0.2
Milk pudding, made with whole milk	129	4.3
Milk, Channel Island, semi-skimmed, UHT	47	1.6
Milk, Channel Island, whole, pasteurised	78	5.1
Milk, Channel Island, whole, pasteurised, summer	78	5.1
Milk, Channel Island, whole, pasteurised, winter	78	5.1

Calories measured in kcal per 100g/100ml *Fat measured as a % of 100g/100ml*

Food	CALORIES	FAT
Milk, condensed, skimmed, sweetened	267	0.2
Milk, condensed, whole, sweetened	333	10.1
Milk, dried, skimmed	348	0.6
Milk, dried, skimmed, with vegetable fat	487	25.9
Milk, evaporated, whole	151	9.4
Milk, flavoured	68	1.5
Milk, flavoured, banana, Nesquik, made with semi-skimmed milk (Nestlé)	132	3.8
Milk, flavoured, banana, Nesquik, made with whole milk (Nestlé)	169	7.9
Milk, flavoured, chocolate, Nesquik, made with semi-skimmed milk (Nestlé)	135	4.1

Calories measured in kcal per 100g/100ml *Fat measured as a % of 100g/100ml*

Food	CALORIES	FAT
Milk, flavoured, chocolate, Nesquik, made with whole milk (Nestlé)	172	8.2
Milk, flavoured, banana, Nesquik, ready to drink (Nestlé)	68	1.8
Milk, goats, pasteurised	60	3.5
Milk, semi-skimmed, pasteurised	46	1.6
Milk, semi-skimmed, pasteurised, fortified plus SMP	51	1.6
Milk, semi-skimmed, UHT	46	1.7
Milk, skimmed, pasteurised	33	0.1
Milk, skimmed, pasteurised, fortified, plus SMP	39	0.1
Milk, skimmed, UHT, fortified	35	0.2
Milk, soya, flavoured	40	1.7
Milk, soya, plain	32	1.9

Calories measured in kcal per 100g/100ml *Fat measured as a % of 100g/100ml*

Food	CALORIES	FAT
Milk, whole, pasteurised	66	3.9
Milk, whole, pasteurised, summer	66	3.9
Milk, whole, pasteurised, winter	66	3.9
Milk, whole, sterilised	66	3.9
Milkshake powder, made with semi-skimmed milk	69	1.6
Milkshake powder, made with whole milk	87	3.7
Mincemeat	274	4.3
Mint jelly (Colman's)	363	0.1
Moussaka	184	13.6
Mousse, chocolate	139	5.4
Mousse, Aero Mousses, all flavours (Chambourcy)	211	8.6
Mousse, fruit	137	5.7
Mushrooms, boiled	11	0.3

Calories measured in kcal per 100g/100ml *Fat measured as a % of 100g/100ml*

Food	CALORIES	FAT
Mushrooms, fried in blended oil	157	16.2
Mushrooms, fried in corn oil	157	16.2
Mushrooms, fried in butter	157	16.2
Mushrooms, raw	13	0.5
Mussels, boiled	87	2.0
Mustard and cress, raw	13	0.6
Mustard, Dijon (Colman's)	153	10.5
Mustard, English (Colman's)	185	9.0
Mustard, French (Colman's)	103	6.5
Mustard, German (Colman's)	97	7.0
Mustard, smooth	139	8.2
Mustard, wholegrain	140	10.2
Mustard, wholegrain (Colman's)	172	11.0
Mustard powder	452	28.7
Mutton biriani	276	16.9

Calories measured in kcal per 100g/100ml *Fat measured as a % of 100g/100ml*

Food	CALORIES	FAT
Mutton curry	374	33.4
Nectarines	40	0.1
Noodles, egg, boiled	62	0.5
Nutmeg, ground	N	36.3
Nuts, almonds	612	55.8
Nuts, Brazil	682	68.2
Nuts, cashew, roasted and salted	611	50.9
Nuts, chestnuts	170	2.7
Nuts, coconut, creamed block	669	68.8
Nuts, coconut, desiccated (Holland & Barrett)	605	63.0
Nuts, hazelnuts	650	63.5
Nuts, macadamia, salted	748	77.6
Nuts, mixed	607	54.1
Nuts, peanuts, dry roasted	589	49.8
Nuts, peanuts, plain	564	46.1

Calories measured in kcal per 100g/100ml *Fat measured as a % of 100g/100ml*

Food	CALORIES	FAT
Nuts, peanuts, roasted and salted	602	53.0
Nuts, pecan	689	70.1
Nuts, pine nuts	688	68.6
Nuts, pistachio, weighed with shells	331	30.5
Nuts, walnuts	688	68.5
Oatmeal	375	9.2
Oil, coconut	899	99.9
Oil, cod liver	899	99.9
Oil, corn	899	99.9
Oil, cottonseed	899	99.9
Oil, olive	899	99.9
Oil, peanut	899	99.9
Oil, rapeseed	899	99.9
Oil, safflower	899	99.9
Oil, sesame	881	99.7

Calories measured in kcal per 100g/100ml *Fat measured as a % of 100g/100ml*

Food	CALORIES	FAT
Oil, soya	899	99.9
Oil, sunflower	899	99.9
Oil, vegetable	899	99.9
Oil, wheatgerm	899	99.9
Okra, boiled	28	0.9
Okra, stir-fried in corn oil	269	26.1
Olives, in brine	103	11.0
Omelette, cheese	266	22.6
Omelette, plain	191	16.4
Onions, boiled	17	0.1
Onions, fried in blended oil	164	11.2
Onions, fried in corn oil	164	11.2
Onions, fried in lard	164	11.2
Onions, pickled	24	0.2
Onions, raw	36	0.2
Onions, silverskin	15	0.1
Oranges	37	0.1

Calories measured in kcal per 100g/100ml *Fat measured as a % of 100g/100ml*

Food	CALORIES	FAT
Oxtail, stewed	243	13.4
Pancake roll	217	12.5
Pancakes, savoury, made with whole milk	273	17.5
Pancakes, Scotch	292	11.7
Pancakes, sweet, made with whole milk	301	16.2
Parsnip, boiled	66	1.2
Partridge, roast, meat only	212	7.2
Passion fruit	36	0.4
Pastry, flaky, cooked	560	40.6
Pastry, shortcrust, cooked	521	32.3
Pastry, wholemeal, cooked	499	32.9
Pâté, beef (Shippams)	203	14.2
Pâté, chicken (Shippams)	232	18.5
Pâté, chicken and ham (Shippams)	227	17.7

Calories measured in kcal per 100g/100ml *Fat measured as a % of 100g/100ml*

Food	CALORIES	FAT
Pâté, crab (Shippams)	97	3.2
Pâté, ham (Shippams)	180	10.9
Pâté, ham and beef (Shippams)	189	13.5
Pâté, herb (Tartex)	231	19.0
Pâté, herb and garlic (Tartex)	231	19.0
Pâté, liver	316	28.9
Pâté, liver and bacon (Shippams)	188	12.5
Pâté, low-fat	191	12.0
Pâté, pepper (Tartex)	241	18.4
Paw-paw, canned in juice	65	Tr
Paw-paw, raw	36	0.1
Peaches, canned in juice	39	Tr
Peaches, canned in syrup	55	Tr
Peaches, canned in syrup (Del Monte)	58	0.1

Calories measured in kcal per 100g/100ml *Fat measured as a % of 100g/100ml*

Food	CALORIES	FAT
Peaches, raw	33	Tr
Peanut butter	623	53.7
Peanut butter (Sun-pat)	620	50.9
Peanuts and raisins	435	26.0
Peanuts and raisins (Holland & Barrett)	466	31.0
Pears, canned in juice	33	Tr
Pears, canned in syrup	50	Tr
Pears, raw	40	0.1
Peas, boiled	79	1.6
Peas, canned	80	0.9
Peas, frozen, boiled	69	0.9
Peas, mangetout, boiled	26	0.1
Peas, mangetout, stir-fried in blended oil	71	4.8
Peas, mushy, canned	81	0.7
Peas, petit pois, frozen, boiled	49	0.9

Calories measured in kcal per 100g/100ml *Fat measured as a % of 100g/100ml*

Food	CALORIES	FAT
Peas, processed, canned	99	0.7
Peppers, capsicum, green, boiled	18	0.5
Peppers, capsicum, green, raw	15	0.3
Peppers, capsicum, red, boiled	34	0.4
Peppers, capsicum, red, raw	32	0.4
Pheasant, roast, meat only	213	9.3
Pickle, Branston Sandwich (Crosse & Blackwell)	122	0.1
Pickle, lime (Sharwood)	152	3.6
Pickle, Piccalilli (Heinz)	89	0.3
Pickle, sweet	134	0.3
Pickle, sweet (Burgess)	167	Tr
Pickle, sweet (Heinz)	114	27.3
Pickle, tomato (Heinz)	105	0.2
Pigeon, roast, meat only	230	13.2
Pilchards	126	5.4

Calories measured in kcal per 100g/100ml *Fat measured as a % of 100g/100ml*

Food	CALORIES	FAT
Pineapple, canned in juice	47	Tr
Pineapple, canned in syrup	64	Tr
Pineapple, canned in syrup (Del Monte)	58	0.1
Pineapple, raw	41	0.2
Pineapple, rings, canned in natural juice (Libby)	50	Tr
Pineapple, rings, canned in syrup (Libby)	80	Tr
Pizza	235	11.8
Pizza, cheese and onion deep topped slices (McVitie's)	223	8.2
Pizza, cheese and tomato French bread pizza (Heinz)	136	3.9
Pizza, cheese supreme deep pan pizza (McCain)	212	6.3
Pizza, ham and mushroom (McCain)	194	5.7

Calories measured in kcal per 100g/100ml *Fat measured as a % of 100g/100ml*

Food	CALORIES	FAT
Plaice, steamed	93	1.9
Plaice fillets in crumbs, fried	228	13.7
Plaice in batter, fried in blended oil	279	18.0
Plaice in batter, fried in dripping	279	18.0
Plantain, boiled	112	0.2
Plantain, ripe, fried in vegetable oil	267	9.2
Plums, canned in syrup	59	Tr
Plums, raw	36	0.1
Plums, stewed, weighed with stones	29	0.1
Plums, stewed with sugar, weighed with stones	75	0.1
Polony	281	21.1
Popcorn, candied	480	20.0

Calories measured in kcal per 100g/100ml *Fat measured as a % of 100g/100ml*

Food	CALORIES	FAT
Popcorn, plain	592	42.8
Poppadams, fried in vegetable oil	369	16.9
Pork, belly rashers, grilled	398	34.8
Pork, chops, loin, grilled	332	24.2
Pork, chops, loin, grilled, lean only	226	10.7
Pork, cooked	619	62.2
Pork, leg, roast	286	19.8
Pork, leg, roast, lean only	185	6.9
Pork, trotters and tails, salted, boiled	280	22.3
Pork pie	376	27.0
Potato, instant powder mix made with water	57	0.1
Potato, instant powder mix made with whole milk	76	1.2
Potato crisps	546	37.6

Calories measured in kcal per 100g/100ml *Fat measured as a % of 100g/100ml*

Food	CALORIES	FAT
Potato crisps, low-fat	456	21.5
Potato croquettes, fried in blended oil	214	13.1
Potato hoops	523	32.0
Potato salad (Heinz)	177	11.0
Potato waffles, frozen, cooked	200	8.2
Potatoes, new, boiled	75	0.3
Potatoes, new, boiled in skins	66	0.3
Potatoes, new, canned	63	0.1
Potatoes, old, baked, flesh and skin	136	0.2
Potatoes, old, baked, flesh only	77	0.1
Potatoes, old, boiled	72	0.1
Potatoes, old, mashed with butter	104	4.3
Potatoes, old, mashed with margarine	104	4.3

Calories measured in kcal per 100g/100ml *Fat measured as a % of 100g/100ml*

Food	CALORIES	FAT
Potatoes, old, roast in lard	149	4.5
Potatoes, roast in blended oil	149	4.5
Potatoes, roast in corn oil	149	4.5
Prawns, boiled	107	1.8
Prunes, canned in juice	79	0.2
Prunes, canned in syrup	90	0.2
Prunes, ready-to-eat	141	0.4
Pumpkin, boiled	13	0.3
Quiche, cheese and egg	314	22.2
Quiche, cheese and egg, wholemeal	308	22.4
Quorn, myco-protein (Marlow Foods)	86	3.5
Rabbit, stewed, meat only	179	7.7
Radish, red, raw	12	0.2
Raisins	272	0.4
Raspberries, canned in syrup	88	0.1

Calories measured in kcal per 100g/100ml *Fat measured as a % of 100g/100ml*

Food	CALORIES	FAT
Raspberries, raw	25	0.3
Ravioli, in tomato sauce	70	2.2
Rhubarb, canned in syrup	31	Tr
Rhubarb, raw	7	0.1
Rhubarb, stewed	7	0.1
Rhubarb, stewed with sugar	48	0.1
Rice, basmati (Uncle Ben's)	343	0.6
Rice, brown, boiled	141	1.1
Rice, creamed (Ambrosia)	90.0	1.6
Rice, creamed, low-fat (Ambrosia)	76	0.8
Rice, egg-fried	208	10.6
Rice, ground (Whitworths)	361	1.0
Rice, savoury	142	3.5
Rice, white, boiled	138	1.3
Rice pudding, canned	89	2.5
Rice pudding, creamed (Libby)	88	1.6

Calories measured in kcal per 100g/100ml *Fat measured as a % of 100g/100ml*

Food	CALORIES	FAT
Rice pudding, low-fat, no added sugar (Heinz)	73	1.5
Risotto, plain	224	9.3
Roe, cod, hard, fried	202	11.9
Roe, herring, soft, fried	244	15.8
Saith, steamed	99	0.6
Salad cream	348	31.0
Salad cream, light (Heinz)	235	20.5
Salad cream, reduced calorie	194	17.2
Salad cream, reduced calorie (Crosse & Blackwell)	371	34.0
Salad dressing, cocktail (Crosse & Blackwell)	147	9.0
Salad dressing, French	651	72.1
Salad dressing, low-fat (Heinz)	107	4.4
Salad dressing, Original French (Kraft)	497	55.0

Calories measured in kcal per 100g/100ml *Fat measured as a % of 100g/100ml*

Food	CALORIES	FAT
Salad dressing, vinaigrette, fat-free (Kraft)	40	Tr
Salad dressing, vinaigrette, low-fat (Heinz)	31	0
Salami	490	45.1
Salmon, canned	155	8.2
Salmon, smoked	142	4.5
Salmon, steamed	197	13.0
Salt, block	0	0
Salt, table	0	0
Samosas, meat	592	56.0
Samosas, vegetable	472	41.8
Sandwich spread (Heinz)	220	12.6
Sardines, canned in oil	217	13.6
Sardines, canned in tomato sauce	177	11.6
Satsumas	36	0.1

Calories measured in kcal per 100g/100ml *Fat measured as a % of 100g/100ml*

Food	CALORIES	FAT
Sauce, apple (Heinz)	61.0	0.2
Sauce, apple sauce mix (Knorr)	379	3.3
Sauce, barbecue	75	1.8
Sauce, bolognese	145	11.1
Sauce, bolognese, cooked with mushrooms (Buitoni)	60	0.9
Sauce, bread, made with semi-skimmed milk	93	3.1
Sauce, bread, made with whole milk	110	5.1
Sauce, brown	99	0
Sauce, brown (Daddies)	87.0	0.3
Sauce, cheese, made with semi-skimmed milk	179	12.6
Sauce, cheese, made with whole milk	197	14.6

Calories measured in kcal per 100g/100ml *Fat measured as a % of 100g/100ml*

Food	CALORIES	FAT
Sauce, chilli (Heinz)	104	0.2
Sauce, cook-in-sauces	43	0.8
Sauce, cranberry (Baxters)	126	0
Sauce, curry, canned	78	5.0
Sauce, garlic (Lee & Perrins)	322	30.0
Sauce, ginger (Lea & Perrins)	110	0.5
Sauce, horseradish	153	8.4
Sauce, mint	87	Tr
Sauce, mint (Coleman's)	122	0.1
Sauce, onion, made with semi-skimmed milk	86	5.0
Sauce, onion, made with whole milk	99	6.5
Sauce, pasta	47	1.5
Sauce, pasta, with mushrooms (Dolmio)	36	Tr
Sauce, pasta, with spicy peppers (Dolmio)	36	Tr

Calories measured in kcal per 100g/100ml *Fat measured as a % of 100g/100ml*

Food	CALORIES	FAT
Sauce, parsley (Coleman's)	320	1.7
Sauce, prawn cocktail (Burgess)	340	29.5
Sauce, seafood (Colman's)	395	37.0
Sauce, soy	64	0
Sauce, sweet and sour (Campbell's)	70	0.3
Sauce, tartare (Coleman's)	273	21.0
Sauce, tomato	91	5.5
Sauce, tomato (Crosse & Blackwell)	125	0.1
Sauce, tomato (Daddies)	118	0.6
Sauce, tomato (Heinz)	101	0.1
Sauce, tomato (HP)	119	1.0
Sauce, white, made with semi-skimmed milk	128	7.8
Sauce, white, made with whole milk	150	10.3

Calories measured in kcal per 100g/100ml *Fat measured as a % of 100g/100ml*

Food	CALORIES	FAT
Sauce, white, sweet, made with semi-skimmed milk	150	7.2
Sauce, white, sweet, made with whole milk	170	9.5
Sausage roll, flaky pastry	477	36.4
Sausage roll, short pastry	459	31.9
Sausages, beef, fried	269	18.0
Sausages, beef, grilled	265	17.3
Sausages, low-fat, fried	211	13.0
Sausages, low-fat, grilled	229	13.8
Sausages, pork, fried	317	24.5
Sausages, pork, grilled	318	24.6
Saveloy	262	20.5
Scampi, in breadcrumbs, frozen, fried	316	17.6
Scones, fruit	316	9.8
Scones, plain	362	14.6
Scones, wholemeal	326	14.4

Calories measured in kcal per 100g/100ml *Fat measured as a % of 100g/100ml*

Food	CALORIES	FAT
Semolina, creamed (Ambrosia)	82	1.7
Semolina pudding (Whitworths)	350	1.8
Sesame seeds	598	58.0
Shepherd's pie	118	6.2
Shrimps, canned	94	1.2
Shrimps, frozen, without shells	73	0.8
Skate in batter, fried	199	12.1
Soup, asparagus, cream of (Baxters)	66	4.9
Soup, asparagus, cream of (Campbell's)	43	2.7
Soup, asparagus, cream of (Heinz)	43	2.8
Soup, beef (Heinz)	400	1.8
Soup, beef and vegetable (Heinz)	37	0.6

Calories measured in kcal per 100g/100ml *Fat measured as a % of 100g/100ml*

Food	CALORIES	FAT
Soup, celery, cream of (Heinz)	43	2.8
Soup, chicken (Heinz)	22	1.1
Soup, chicken, cream of, canned	58	3.8
Soup, chicken, cream of, canned, condensed	49	3.6
Soup, chicken, low-calorie (Knorr)	303	1.1
Soup, chicken and leek (Campbell's)	50	3.5
Soup, chicken and mushroom (Heinz)	38	2.2
Soup, chicken and vegetable (Heinz)	41	1.0
Soup, chicken noodle (Heinz)	18	0.2
Soup, chicken noodle, dried, ready-to-serve	20	0.3
Soup, French onion (Knorr)	311	4.5

Calories measured in kcal per 100g/100ml *Fat measured as a % of 100g/100ml*

Food	CALORIES	FAT
Soup, instant powder, made with water	64	2.3
Soup, leek, cream of (Baxters)	45	2.4
Soup, leek and potato (Batchelors)	47	3.0
Soup, lentil	99	3.8
Soup, low-calorie, canned	20	0.2
Soup, minestrone, dried, ready-to-serve	23	0.7
Soup, mushroom (Heinz)	24	0.6
Soup, mushroom, cream of, canned	53	3.8
Soup, onion, cream of (Campbell's)	44	2.8
Soup, oxtail, canned	44	1.7
Soup, oxtail, dried, ready-to-serve	27	0.8

Calories measured in kcal per 100g/100ml *Fat measured as a % of 100g/100ml*

Food	CALORIES	FAT
Soup, pea and ham (Heinz)	54	1.1
Soup, potato and leek (Heinz)	34	0.6
Soup, prawn, cream of (Campbell's)	540	3.6
Soup, tomato (Batchelors)	60	3.3
Soup, tomato, creamed (Crosse & Blackwell)	76	3.7
Soup, tomato, cream of, canned	55	3.3
Soup, tomato, cream of, canned, condensed	123	6.8
Soup, tomato, dried, ready-to-serve	31	0.5
Soup, tomato, reduced calorie (Batchelors)	27	0.4
Soup, vegetable, canned	37	0.7
Soup, vegetable (Crosse & Blackwell)	39	0.7
Soup, vegetable (Heinz)	24	0.2

Calories measured in kcal per 100g/100ml *Fat measured as a % of 100g/100ml*

Food	CALORIES	FAT
Soup, vegetable (Knorr)	290	2.7
Soup, vegetable, low-calorie Knorr)	296	1.9
Spaghetti, Aladdin spaghetti shapes in tomato sauce (Heinz)	67	0.4
Spaghetti, alphabet, in tomato sauce (Crosse & Blackwell)	60	0.4
Spaghetti, in tomato sauce	64	0.4
Spaghetti, in tomato sauce (Heinz)	64	0.4
Spaghetti, in tomato sauce, no added sugar (Heinz)	51	0.4
Spaghetti, in tomato sauce with sausages (Heinz)	108	4.7
Spaghetti, white, boiled	104	0.7
Spaghetti, wholemeal, boiled	113	0.9
Spaghetti bolognese (Heinz)	97	2.6

Calories measured in kcal per 100g/100ml *Fat measured as a % of 100g/100ml*

Food	CALORIES	FAT
Spaghetti hoops (Heinz)	61	0.4
Spinach, boiled	19	0.8
Sponge pudding	340	16.3
Spring greens, boiled	20	0.7
Spring onions, raw	23	0.5
Stock cubes, beef (CPC Foods)	181	4.2
Stock cubes, beef (Knorr)	318	17.8
Stock cubes, chicken (Brooke Bond)	252	4.0
Stock cubes, chicken (CPC Foods)	195	4.1
Stock cubes, chicken (Knorr)	316	17.6
Stock cubes, fish (Knorr)	299	20.4
Stock cubes, ham (Knorr)	261	16.5
Stock cubes, lamb (Knorr)	326	20.0
Stock cubes, pork (Knorr)	355	23.0
Stock cubes, vegetable (Knorr)	328	19.0

Calories measured in kcal per 100g/100ml *Fat measured as a % of 100g/100ml*

Food	CALORIES	FAT
Strawberries, canned in syrup	65	Tr
Strawberries, raw	27	0.1
Stuffing, sage and onion	231	14.8
Stuffing mix, made with water	97	1.5
Suet, shredded	826	86.7
Sugar, brown, soft (Tate & Lyle)	386	0
Sugar, demerara	394	0
Sugar, icing (Tate & Lyle)	398	0
Sugar, white	394	0
Sultanas	275	0.4
Sunflower seeds	581	47.5
Swede, boiled	11	0.1
Sweetbread, lamb, fried	230	14.6
Sweetcorn, baby, canned	23	0.4
Sweetcorn, kernels, canned	122	1.2
Sweetcorn, on the cob	66	1.4

Calories measured in kcal per 100g/100ml *Fat measured as a % of 100g/100ml*

Food	CALORIES	FAT
Sweet potato, boiled	84	0.3
Sweets, boiled	327	Tr
Sweets, chewing gum, Orbit Fruit (Wrigley)	180	0
Sweets, chewing gum, Orbit Peppermint (Wrigley)	190	0
Sweets, chewing gum, Orbit Spearmint (Wrigley)	195	0
Sweets, liquorice allsorts	313	2.2
Sweets, Opal Fruits (Mars)	411	7.6
Sweets, pastilles	253	0
Sweets, pear drops (Cravens)	386	0
Sweets, peppermints	392	0.7
Sweets, Polo Mints (Nestlé)	404	1.1
Sweets, sherbert lemons (Cravens)	423	7.4
Sweets, Softmints (Trebor Bassett)	16	0.2

Calories measured in kcal per 100g/100ml *Fat measured as a % of 100g/100ml*

Food	CALORIES	FAT
Sweets, toffee	430	17.2
Sweets, Tunes (Mars)	392	0
Sweets, Turkish delight	295	0
Sweets, Turkish delight (Cadbury)	524	30.0
Syrup, golden	298	0
Tahini paste	607	58.9
Tangerines	35	0.1
Tapioca, creamed (Ambrosia)	81	1.6
Taramasalata	446	46.4
Tea, Indian, infusion	Tr	Tr
Teacakes, toasted	329	8.3
Tofu, soya bean, steamed	73	4.2
Tofu, soya bean, steamed, fried	261	17.7
Tomato ketchup	98	Tr
Tomato purée	68	0.2

Calories measured in kcal per 100g/100ml *Fat measured as a % of 100g/100ml*

Food	CALORIES	FAT
Tomatoes, canned, chopped (Napolina)	15	Tr
Tomatoes, canned whole	16	0.1
Tomatoes, fried in blended oil	91	7.7
Tomatoes, fried in corn oil	91	7.7
Tomatoes, fried in lard	91	7.7
Tomatoes, grilled	49	0.9
Tomatoes, raw	17	0.3
Tongue, canned	213	16.5
Tongue, lamb, raw	193	14.6
Tongue, ox, boiled	293	23.9
Tongue, ox, raw, pickled	220	17.5
Tongue, sheep, stewed	289	24.0
Tortilla chips	459	22.6
Treacle, black	257	0
Treacle tart	368	14.1
Trifle	160	6.3

Calories measured in kcal per 100g/100ml *Fat measured as a % of 100g/100ml*

Food	CALORIES	FAT
Trifle, peach (St Ivel)	152	5.4
Trifle, raspberry (St Ivel)	153	5.4
Trifle, strawberry (St Ivel)	149	5.4
Trifle, strawberry, luxury (St Ivel)	167	8.1
Trifle, with fresh cream	166	9.2
Tripe, dressed	60	2.5
Tripe, dressed, stewed	100	4.5
Trout, brown, steamed	135	4.5
Tuna, canned in brine	99	0.6
Tuna, canned in oil	189	9.0
Turkey, roast, dark meat	148	4.1
Turkey, roast, light meat	132	1.4
Turkey, roast, meat and skin	171	6.5
Turkey, roast, meat only	140	2.7
Turnip, boiled	12	0.2
Twiglets (Jacob's)	395	11.1

Calories measured in kcal per 100g/100ml *Fat measured as a % of 100g/100ml*

Food	CALORIES	FAT
Tzatziki	66	4.9
Veal cutlet, fried in vegetable oil	215	8.1
Veal fillet, roast	230	11.5
Vegetables, mixed, frozen, boiled	42	0.5
Venison, roast	198	6.4
Vinegar	4	0
Vinegar, cider (Holland & Barrett)	1.8	0
Vinegar, malt (HP)	4.6	0
Vinaigrette dressing, fat-free (Kraft)	40	Tr
Vinaigrette dressing, French (Kraft)	424	44.0
Vinaigrette dressing, low-fat (Heinz)	31	0
Vinaigrette dressing, oil-free (Crosse & Blackwell)	13	0.2

Calories measured in kcal per 100g/100ml *Fat measured as a % of 100g/100ml*

Food	CALORIES	FAT
Wafers, ice cream	342	0.7
Water	0	0
Watercress, raw	22	1.0
Wheat, brown	323	1.8
Wheat, white, breadmaking	341	1.4
Wheat, white, plain	341	1.3
Wheat, white, self-raising	330	1.2
Wheat, wholemeal	310	2.2
Whelks, boiled, weighed with shell	14	0.3
White pudding	450	31.8
Whitebait, fried	525	47.5
Whiting, in crumbs, fried	191	10.3
Whiting, steamed	92	0.9
Winkles, boiled, weighed with shell	14	0.3
Yam, boiled	133	0.3

Calories measured in kcal per 100g/100ml *Fat measured as a % of 100g/100ml*

Food	CALORIES	FAT
Yeast, bakers', compressed	53	0.4
Yeast, dried	169	1.5
Yoghurt, black cherry (Ski)	95	1.1
Yoghurt, black cherry (St Ivel)	42	0.1
Yoghurt, drinking	62	Tr
Yoghurt, forest fruits (St Ivel)	41	0
Yoghurt, Greek, cows	115	9.1
Yoghurt, Greek, sheep	106	7.5
Yoghurt, Greek style, natural (St Ivel)	153	10.4
Yoghurt, low-calorie	41	0.2
Yoghurt, low-fat, flavoured	90	0.9
Yoghurt, low-fat, fruit	90	0.7
Yoghurt, low-fat, natural (Holland & Barrett)	65	1.0
Yoghurt, low-fat, natural (St Ivel)	64	1.2

Calories measured in kcal per 100g/100ml *Fat measured as a % of 100g/100ml*

Food	CALORIES	FAT
Yoghurt, low-fat, plain	56	0.8
Yoghurt, orange, (Ski)	88	0.7
Yoghurt, peach (Ski)	94	1.1
Yoghurt, peach melba (St Ivel)	41	0.1
Yoghurt, pineapple (Ski)	96	1.1
Yoghurt, raspberry (St Ivel)	41	0.1
Yoghurt, raspberry (Ski)	94	1.1
Yoghurt, raspberry, low-fat (Holland & Barrett)	83	0.8
Yoghurt, rhubarb (St Ivel)	40	0.1
Yoghurt, soya	72	4.2
Yoghurt, strawberry (St Ivel)	41	0.1
Yoghurt, strawberry cream (St Ivel Shape)	41	0.1
Yoghurt, strawberry, low-fat (Holland & Barrett)	83	0.8
Yoghurt, vanilla (St Ivel)	40	0.1

Calories measured in kcal per 100g/100ml *Fat measured as a % of 100g/100ml*

Food	CALORIES	FAT
Yoghurt, whole milk, fruit	105	2.8
Yoghurt, whole milk, plain	79	3.0
Yorkshire pudding	208	9.9

Calories measured in kcal per 100g/100ml *Fat measured as a % of 100g/100ml*

Calorie Counter – Alcoholic Drinks

Alcoholic drinks	CALORIES	FAT
Advocaat	272	6.3
Beer, bitter, canned	32	Tr
Beer, draught	32	Tr
Beer, keg	31	Tr
Beer, mild draught	25	Tr
Brown ale, bottled	28	Tr
Cherry brandy	255	0
Cider, dry	36	0
Cider, sweet	42	0
Cider, vintage	101	0
Curaçao	311	0
Lager, bottled	29	Tr
Pale ale, bottled	32	Tr
Port	157	0
Sherry, dry	116	0
Sherry, medium	118	0
Sherry, sweet	136	0

Calories measured in kcal per 100g/100ml *Fat measured as a % of 100g/100ml*

Alcoholic drinks	CALORIES	FAT
Spirits, 40% volume	222	0
Stout, bottled	37	Tr
Stout, extra	39	Tr
Strong ale	72	Tr
Vermouth, dry	118	0
Vermouth, sweet	151	0
Wine, red	68	0
Wine, rosé	71	0
Wine, white, dry	66	0
Wine, white, medium	75	0
Wine, white, sparkling	76	0
Wine, white, sweet	94	0

Recipes

Here are some easy-to-prepare meals to help you start planning your weekly menus. Use the Calorie and fat content information to plan your Calorie and fat intake for each day. When you have collected a good range of recipes use the menu planner at the end of the book to plan your favourite meals for a week or more. Your new routine will help you to control your eating habits and to buy the ingredients you really need when you go shopping.

BREAKFAST

Breakfast cereal

Calories per serving: 54
Fat per serving: 0.7 g

40 g high-fibre cereal, such as All-Bran, made with 50 ml skimmed milk

Home-made muesli

Calories per serving: 160
Fat per serving: 6 g

4 tbsp rolled porridge oats
2 tbsp low-fat yoghurt
1 tbsp chopped hazelnuts
1 tsp lemon juice
50 g apple
6 tsp water

- Stir the oats, yoghurt, water and lemon juice in a large bowl until creamy.
- Add the apple and sprinkle with the chopped nuts.

Fruity yoghurt (serves 2)
Calories per serving: 165
Fat per serving: 0.8 g

100 g dried mixed fruit (such as apples, apricots, pears, prunes)
1/4 tsp allspice
1/4 tsp cinnamon
100 ml water
1 tbsp plain, low-fat yoghurt

- Soak the fruits and spices in the water overnight.
- Serve cold, adding 1 tablespoonful of plain, low-fat yoghurt.

Home-made muffins and fruit (serves 2)
Calories per muffin: 135
Fat per muffin: 4 g

25 g rolled oats
12 g plain flour
12 g buckwheat flour
18 ml apple juice
12 ml skimmed milk
1/2 egg
1/4 tbsp corn oil
1/4 eating apple, finely chopped
12 g very soft fruits (berry fruits such as blackcurrants work well)
1/4 tbsp sugar
1/4 tsp baking powder
Pinch of ground cinnamon

- Lightly grease a muffin tin base with a little cooking oil.
- Heat oven to 200 °C, 400 °F, Gas Mark 6.
- In one bowl combine the milk, apple juice, egg and oil, in another, all the dry ingredients.
- To the wet mixture add the apple and fruits.
- Fold the dry ingredients into the wet mixture.
- Put the mixture into the muffin tins and bake until the muffins are golden and risen (about 18 minutes).

LUNCH

Green salad with French dressing (serves 2)

Calories per serving (using 2 tsp dressing): 260

Fat per serving: 12.9 g

For the salad:

12 g salad rocket

Handful of watercress and lettuce leaves

Few spring onions

25 g bean sprouts

25 g sliced mushrooms

1/8 cauliflower

For 142ml of dressing:

87 ml sunflower oil

50 ml lemon juice

1/4 tsp mustard

1 clove garlic, crushed

Pinch root ginger

Pinch ground pepper

- Wash and clean the vegetables.
- Tear the lettuce into small pieces and finely chop the watercress stalks and onions.
- Break the cauliflower into small florets.
- Put all salad dressing ingredients into a glass bottle or jar. Shake well.
- Toss each salad portion in two teaspoonfuls of dressing.

Green bean and bacon salad (serves 2)

Calories per serving: 150

Fat per serving: 6.4 g

For the salad:

225 g green beans

2 rashers lean bacon

1/2 small onion

1/2 red pepper

For the dressing:

75 ml plain yoghurt

1/2 tbsp olive oil

1/2 tbsp lemon juice

1/2 clove garlic

1 tbsp chopped chives

Pinch black pepper

- Trim and slice the beans. Steam until slightly tender.
- Trim any fat off the bacon and grill. Chop into small pieces.
- Finely chop the onion and red pepper and mix with the beans and bacon.
- Mix all dressing ingredients together.
- Crush the clove of garlic and mix with other dressing ingredients.
- Toss salad in the dressing.

Broccoli soup (serves 2)

Calories per serving: 165

Fat per serving: 2.5 g

162 g broccoli

225 g potatoes

1/2 small onion

137 ml semi-skimmed milk

Pinch salt

350 ml chicken or vegetable stock
Pinch black pepper

- Cut broccoli into small florets.
- Peel potatoes and cut into chunks.
- Put everything into a saucepan and simmer for 25 minutes.
- When cooked, liquidize.
- Return to pan and reheat if necessary.
- Season and serve.

Tuna and pasta salad (serves 2)
Calories per serving: 405
Fat per serving: 9 g

200 g tuna (in brine if possible)
75 g dry pasta shapes
50 g tinned butter beans or kidney beans
50 g tinned sweetcorn
25 g raisins
2 sticks celery
1 apple
5 tbsp oil-free French dressing
1 tbsp olive oil
Pinch caster sugar

- Mix the oil-free dressing with the olive oil and sugar.
- Cook and drain the pasta.
- Drain the tuna and add to the pasta.
- Chop the celery and apple.
- Mix into the pasta and tuna together with the beans, sweetcorn and raisins.
- Add the dressing and mix well.

Pepperoni salad (serves 2)
Calories per serving: 185
Fat per serving: 1.9 g

12 g pepperoni, sliced
112 g broad beans, shelled
112 g green beans, sliced
225 g new potatoes
112 g mixed salad leaves
½ small red onion
1½ tbsp low-fat yogurt
1½ tbsp parsley leaves
Drop of Tabasco sauce

- Cook potatoes.
- Add beans, cover and cook for three minutes. Drain.
- Mix in yogurt and Tabasco sauce and leave to cool.
- Chop parsley. Mix in to potatoes with pepperoni and red onion.
- Serve on a green salad.

DINNER

Lamb Casserole (serves 2)
Calories per serving: 340
Fat per serving: 11 g

125 g lean lamb
75 g dry brown lentils
200 g canned chopped tomatoes
1 onion
2 medium carrots
1 bay leaf
1 tsp rosemary
150 ml meat or vegetable stock
Pinch salt and pepper
1 stick celery

- Cube the lamb and brown over a gentle heat.
- Chop the onions, carrots and celery and add to the lamb along with all the other ingredients.
- Cover and simmer for 1½ hours. Halfway through cooking, stir and add more stock if necessary.
- Season before serving.

Sautéed cod with tomatoes (serves 2)

Calories per serving: 200

Fat per serving: 2.5 g

2 cod fillets
2 tomatoes
2 shallots
½ tbsp low-calorie mayonnaise
½ tbsp wholemeal flour
3 tbsp fish stock
Pinch salt
Pinch pepper
A little sunflower oil

- Finely chop the shallots.
- De-seed and chop tomatoes.
- Simmer shallots and tomatoes in stock and seasoning for 30 minutes.
- Blend mixture in a food processor then return to pan to keep warm.
- Combine mustard and mayonnaise.
- Coat fish with mayonnaise mixture then dip in flour.
- Sauté fish in a little sunflower oil, for 10–15 minutes, turning once.
- Serve with the tomato sauce.

Fish-stuffed jacket potatoes (serves 2)
Calories per serving: 279
Fat per serving: 6 g

2 large potatoes	1 tbsp skimmed milk
175 g cooked fish	1 tbsp parley
90 g cheddar cheese	Pinch salt
1 clove garlic	Pinch ground pepper

- Bake the potatoes. Cut lengthwise and remove flesh. Mash the flesh with 60 g cheese.
- Chop the garlic and parsley. Add to the potato mixture along with the milk. Mix to a smooth consistency.
- Remove any skin and bones from the fish. Flake it and add to the potato mixture.
- Season with salt and pepper and return the entire mixture to the potato jackets.
- Sprinkle with the remaining cheese. Bake at 400 °F, 200 °C, Gas Mark 6.

Grilled salmon steaks (serves 2)
Calories per serving: 315
Fat per serving: 24 g

2 salmon steaks	1 1/2 tbsp fresh fennel
1 tbsp olive oil	Juice of 1/2 lemon
1/2 tsp fennel seeds	Lemon wedges to garnish

- To make the marinade, chop the fennel, mix with the olive oil, fennel seeds and lemon juice.

- Coat the steaks with the marinade. Sprinkle with salt and pepper.
- Cover with clingfilm and refrigerate for two hours.
- Then place the steaks in a shallow dish with remaining marinade. Grill for 6–8 minutes until browned, turning once.
- Garnish with lemon wedges and serve with a green salad or steamed vegetables.

Vegetable stir-fry (serves 2)
Calories per serving: 253
Fat per serving: 13.5 g

1 courgette	100 g rice noodles
1/4 red pepper	25 g unsalted cashews
1/4 yellow pepper	1/2 tbsp sesame seeds
100 g mangetout	1/2 tbsp sesame oil
100 g baby sweetcorn	1 tbsp soy sauce

- Wash and prepare the vegetables.
- Heat the oil. Add the vegetables and stir-fry.
- Add cashew nuts and sesame seeds.
- Cook the rice noodles. Add to the vegetables.
- Add soy sauce and serve.

Chicken chilli
Calories per serving: 286
Fat per serving: 10 g

2 chicken breast fillets, skinned, boneless

1 medium onion	1/2 green pepper
200 g tinned chopped tomatoes	1/2 red chilli
100 g cooked red kidney beans	1/2 tbsp flour
125 ml chicken stock	1/2 tbsp corn oil
2 tbsp low-fat yoghurt	1/2 tbsp sweet paprika
1 tbsp chopped parsley	Pinch salt
	Pinch black pepper

- Season the flour with salt and pepper.
- Coat the chicken breasts in the seasoned flour.
- Brown the chicken pieces in the oil then remove from the pan.
- Chop the onion. Seed and chop the green pepper and the red chilli.
- Stir-fry the onion and pepper in the pan for a few minutes.
- Add the chilli and paprika and cook for another minute. If necessary, add a little of the stock.
- Add rest of stock, chopped tomatoes and kidney beans. Cover and simmer for 30 minutes.
- Return chicken to the pan. Simmer for 15 minutes.
- Add salt, pepper and yoghurt.
- Serve garnished with chopped parsley.

Mushroom risotto

Calories per serving: 162

Fat per serving: 7 g

225 g mushrooms (mixed if possible)	112 g wholegrain easy-cook rice

375 ml vegetable stock	1/2 onion
12 g Parmesan cheese	1 tbsp parsley
1 clove garlic	1/2 tbsp olive oil

- Chop the onion and garlic and sauté in the oil until soft.
- Slice the mushrooms. Add to the pan and cook for two minutes.
- Add the rice and cook for two minutes.
- Add 75 ml of the stock and cook over a low heat.
- Stir frequently, gradually adding more stock.
- Chop the parsley. When the rice has absorbed the stock mix in the parsley.
- Serve sprinkled with grated Parmesan cheese.

DESSERT

Hot spicy bananas (serves 2)

Calories per serving: 198

Fat per serving: 11 g

2 large ripe bananas	25 g butter
1/2 tbsp honey	1 tsp allspice

- Bake the bananas in their skins at 180 °C, 350 °F, Gas Mark 4 for 15 minutes. Remove skins.
- Melt butter. Stir in honey and allspice.
- Pour butter mixture over bananas and serve.

Fruit salad (serves 2)
Calories per serving: 90
Fat per serving: Trace

100 g honeydew melon
1/2 grapefruit
1/2 apple
25 g grapes
1 kiwifruit
100 ml apple juice
1/2 dessertspoon sugar
Juice of 1/2 lemon
Few mint leaves

- Wash all fruit. Chop or segment into small pieces.
- Mix together apple juice, lemon juice and sugar.
- Combine fruit with juice mixture. Leave for 1–2 hours in the fridge.
- Serve chilled, garnished with mint.

Strawberry sorbet (serves 2)
Calories per serving: 25
Fat per serving: 0.1 g

150 g strawberries
Juice of 1/2 large orange

- Mix the strawberries and orange juice together until smooth.
- Leave in the freezer for one hour.
- Allow to thaw slightly, then blend well with a metal spoon to break up any ice crystals. Return to the freezer for a minimum of five hours.
- Leave at room temperature for 15 minutes before serving.

Menu Planner

Planning your own menus

Remember that when dieting it is just as important to eat a wide variety of foods in order to gain the amount of protein, carbohydrate, fats, vitamins, minerals and fibre your body needs. Over the course of a week you should aim to eat a range of foods from the four main food groups listed below and on the next two pages. Try to avoid foods that are high in fat or sugar (see the guide on page 11).

Group 1: Bread, cereals and potatoes

Foods in this group include:

- All kinds of bread, bread rolls and chapattis
- Beans and lentils
- Breakfast cereals
- Noodles
- Pasta
- Potatoes
- Rice

These foods should make up the main part of your diet. Choose versions that are high in fibre wherever possible.

Group 2: Fruit and vegetables

Food in this group includes:

- All types of fruit and vegetables, including those in cans as well as fresh varieties.
- Beans and lentils.

It is recommended that you try and eat at least five portions of fruit and vegetables each day.

Group 3: Milk and dairy foods

Food in this group includes:

- Milk
- Cheese
- Yoghurt
- Fromage frais

These foods are high in protein but may also be high in fat so choose low-fat varieties.

Group 4: Meat, fish and alternatives

Food in this group includes:

- All kinds of meat (such as bacon, beef, lamb, pork)
- Meat products (such as beefburgers and sausages)
- All types of poultry (such as chicken and turkey)
- Fish (including canned and frozen fish as well as fresh fish)
- Fish products (such as fish cakes and fish fingers)
- Offal (such as kidney and liver)
- Eggs
- Beans and lentils
- Nuts
- Meat alternatives (such as textured vegetable protein)
- Tofu
- Beancurd
- Soya meats

Sample menu planner

Photocopy the tables on pages 148–154 and fill them in so you have a week or more of daily menus. Check the Calorie and fat contents using the Calorie Counter on page 31.

The foods in the Calorie Counter are listed according to how many Calories and how much fat there is in 100 grams (or 100 millilitres). You will need to weigh the foods that do not come ready labelled in tins (such as fresh meat and fresh fruit and vegetables) in each menu to see how many Calories and how much fat they contain. Then complete the columns for Calorie content and fat content in your menu planner.

Use the sample menu opposite to check that you are filling in your daily menus correctly.

MONDAY	**Calorie content**	**Fat content**
Breakfast		
Glass of unsweetened orange juice	45	0
Scrambled egg on toasted wholemeal bread	55	5.0
1 toasted crumpet with low-fat spread	80	3.0
Snack		
1 pear	70	0.2
Lunch		
Pasta with *a little* pasta sauce	495	6.0
Green salad	20	0
Banana	100	0.3
Snack		
Some grapes	90	0.1
Dinner		
Fatless chicken	200	6.0
Carrots	15	0.2
Broccoli	14	0.4
Low-fat fruit yoghurt	155	1.0
Total daily Calories and fat	1339	22.2

MONDAY

	Calorie content	Fat content
Breakfast		
Snack		
Lunch		
Snack		
Dinner		
Total daily Calories and fat		

TUESDAY

	Calorie content	Fat content
Breakfast		
Snack		
Lunch		
Snack		
Dinner		
Total daily Calories and fat		

WEDNESDAY

	Calorie content	Fat content
Breakfast		
Snack		
Lunch		
Snack		
Dinner		
Total daily Calories and fat		

THURSDAY	Calorie content	Fat content
Breakfast		
Snack		
Lunch		
Snack		
Dinner		
Total daily Calories and fat		

FRIDAY

	Calorie content	Fat content
Breakfast		
Snack		
Lunch		
Snack		
Dinner		
Total daily Calories and fat		

SATURDAY

	Calorie content	Fat content
Breakfast		
Snack		
Lunch		
Snack		
Dinner		
Total daily Calories and fat		

SUNDAY

	Calorie content	Fat content
Breakfast		
Snack		
Lunch		
Snack		
Dinner		
Total daily Calories and fat		